The Comm

The Commonsense Diet

Stop Overthinking, Start Eating

Rujuta Diwekar

juggernaut

JUGGERNAUT BOOKS
C-I-128, First Floor, Sangam Vihar, Near Holi Chowk,
New Delhi 110080, India

First published by Juggernaut Books 2025

Copyright © Rujuta Diwekar 2025

10 9 8 7 6 5 4 3 2 1

P-ISBN: 9789353457501
E-ISBN: 9789353459611

The views and opinions expressed in this book are the author's own. The facts contained herein were reported to be true as on the date of publication by the author to the publishers of the book, and the publishers are not in any way liable for their accuracy or veracity.

All rights reserved. No part of this publication may be reproduced, transmitted, or stored in a retrieval system in any form or by any means without the written permission of the publisher.

Typeset in Adobe Caslon Pro by R. Ajith Kumar, Noida

Printed at Replika Press Pvt. Ltd.

For you Bebo,
And to your patience and wisdom, dear Chiki.

Contents

Foreword by Kareena Kapoor Khan — ix

Introduction — 1

Section 1: Diets Don't Work — **15**

1. 'Sciency' diets — 25
   - 1.1 Playing with nutrients – high protein, low carb, etc. — 25
   - 1.2 Playing with calories – intermittent fasting, skipping meals, etc. — 48
   - 1.3 Playing with single ingredients – sugar, dairy, gluten, etc. — 65
2. Pseudo-cultural trends — 75
   - 2.1 Gut cleanses/detox — 80
   - 2.2 Fasting — 86
   - 2.3 Seeds and spices — 92
   - 2.4 Millets — 96

Section 2: *Ghar Ka Khaana* Works — **107**

3. What is a successful diet? — 109
4. The real meaning of *ghar ka khaana* — 119

5. The three rules of eating *ghar ka khaana*	134
6. What's not *ghar ka khaana*	153
Section 3: Commonsense Eating and Living	**159**
7. The food plan you can depend on	161
8. Tracking progress	174
9. Diet recalls and modifications	184
In Conclusion – A full life	205
Appendices	211
A Note on the Author	223

Foreword

Rujuta and I worked together on *Tashan* and the rest, as they say, is history. It won't be wrong to say that we entirely disrupted the diet scene. *Ghar ka khaana* and bikini bod, once thought of as mutually exclusive, were being spoken about in the same breath.

But now all around me, I find people drowning in trends – from seeds to shots, keto to cleanses. Ironically, all this in the name of health. The foundation of good health, though, is habits; boring – but that is the truth. The habit of eating *ghar ka khaana*, exercising, sleeping early and minding one's own business, serve the best to those interested in health. The rest is just signing up for a longer route in the hope of a short cut.

So, while Rujuta and I started working together in 2007, the things that I have learnt from her continue to stay a part of my life and even my family's. In fact, the reason why I even worked with her was because she didn't have an extreme approach towards fitness. It was a finely calibrated one and I had no intentions of ever giving up on paratha, Sindhi curry and now the pasta that Saif cooks when he's in the mood.

Basically, I come from a line of women who respect and celebrate both food and hard work. My mother would eat rice and fish curry for lunch during her shooting years. My sister, the hardest working girl I know, really knows how to eat. So thankfully, I never saw food as the enemy of fitting into good clothes, having good skin, etc., but rather an accomplice that enables those goals.

Today I have taken on many new roles – producer, homemaker, mother and wife; so I have new appreciation for food. It's not something that helps me with just my waistline but with my bandwidth to pursue it all without running out of fuel. I want to take in the full joy of my boys running in school races, of giving the perfect shot on a film set, of hedging my bets on the best script.

And while I am married to my co-actor from *Tashan*, I am not married to the way I looked in the film. Our bodies, work and relationships, must evolve and stand the test of time. Looking exactly like the way one looked 10 or 20 or 30 years ago is stagnating, not stunning.

An old piece of furniture fades, and pages of an old book, pale. That's where, as Saif says, the beauty lies. In the age and the authenticity it carries with it. To me, health is just that, an act of liberating ourselves from external pretenses. In embracing our age, our bodies, with the flaws, fine lines, hell – even a bit of a paunch. And in surrounding ourselves with people who see us worthy of good food, good roles and good holidays.

Life, after all, is about coming of age. It's about knowing that true joy lies in a hot bowl of khichdi eaten with a crunchy papad while watching your husband read aloud to the boys at bedtime. Looking good is about savouring small joys in real time and not about how thin you looked in reels.

Kareena Kapoor Khan
Mumbai

Introduction

It was 2009 and just a few months after the release of my first book *Don't Lose Your Mind, Lose Your Weight*. I had finished giving a talk in Indore which had about four hundred people in the audience. I was feeling good, very good about myself. As I was making my way towards the car, a lady pulled me by my elbow and asked, '*Yeh wahi hai na, woh* Kareena Kapoor *wali*, don't break my head, just lose weight.'

'Haan,' I nodded, feeling even better *ke faltu mein udne ka nahi.*

The book had intrigued many people. For the first time there was a desi way to lose weight. But more importantly, Kareena Kapoor had lost weight on it, making room for the rich, glam brigade to look at ghee, khichdi, even parathas, with new eyes. *Ghar ka khaana ka* status had gotten elevated; it was now the bikini-bod diet.

I began working in 1999 officially but had been on the gym-aerobics-diet circuit since 1997–98. When I started out, only filmy people were into fitness. After all, looking a certain way mattered to them. And because of their influence, some industrialists too had joined their ranks. But regular people weren't 'into health' the way they are now.

Today, however, everyone wants to look like a movie star. We want a flat stomach if not a six pack, a slim if not skinny body and a sharp if not a taut jawline. Social media is full of 'transformation' pics, and everyone is an expert on health and fitness. The fintech guy, the liver guy, the branding guy – everyone has health advice for you. People put their HbA1c, BMI, resting heart rate on their bio. They even pin posts of their fastest sprint, longest cycling day, heaviest dead lift, whatever.

Appearance

My partner, GP, is from UC Berkeley. One of his closest friends, who lives in the Bay Area, was visiting us. The friend worked with Lyft at the time. He was one of their most senior executives. He told us that one day he was at a meeting with the founder. After it ended, the founder had to go into another meeting so he went to change and came out with his hair ruffled, wearing a crumpled T-shirt and ill-fitting jeans. GP's friend was puzzled. 'Well, that's the "look",' the founder explained. Basically, when you are the start-up guy, the genius working in the garage with a ground-breaking idea that is scalable, etc., you'd better look it. Only then are the VCs going to loosen their purse strings.

> The lesson of this story is simple: We all need to look the part, or at least that's what we are told. If it's a professional requirement, like being formally dressed when you are a doctor or a judge, etc., it's ok. But when you make an external image of an internal state of being, then you goof up. Big time. I am talking about health.

Health is not about maintaining appearances. It's not the six-pack, the weight loss, the skinny jeans or your fasting sugars, running efficiency or sleep score. It's about living a kinder, gentler life. It empowers us to live more freely, openly, fully. When people are scared or shamed into getting 'healthier', it just doesn't work. Fear and shame are the opposite of love. Love can move mountains, and you need that positive force in your life, because building health and staying healthy is a job for a lifetime. This means that it is about monotonous, repetitive, routine habits that you do with a fresh perspective, daily. And you can have that kind of commitment only when there is love.

They say Sachin Tendulkar would be the first one to show up at the nets to practise. His seniority or the stardom he enjoyed or how much he scored in the previous match didn't matter. That's how you get a hundred 100s – keep your head down and bat.

That's also what the legendary basketball player Michael Jordan had said – it's all about practice. If you practice every day, when you get to the moment, you don't have to think about it. Things happen instinctively. It's the same for your health. It will come through like a class act when it really matters, but the everyday practice of it means doing the same old boring stuff, day in, day out.

What's health anyway?

One of my favourite quotes about health comes from the great yoga guru B.K.S. Iyengar. 'Health is where you forget about your body.' I once heard a story that elaborated on this idea. It was 2005. I was sitting on the banks of the Ganga in Rishikesh, listening to Swami Dayananda Saraswati speak. I tend to find *bhashans* too preachy, and the ones that come from swamis can also be very boring. But that day, Swami Dayananda made all of us in the audience laugh and nod in amusement and recognition. I guess this is what it means to be a good speaker: one who knows how to connect. He simplified what others mystified.

Swamiji was talking about meditation, and he acted out the stereotype we all have about it. He closed his eyes, did a mudra with his hands and inhaled and exhaled loudly. The crowd giggled. Rishikesh is full of banners depicting meditation like this – three- to thirty-day courses are available, and even come with a certificate. Meditation, he said, is not what you can see outside but what is happening inside. It isn't what the world sees about you but what you see about the world.

He told us a story. One day he was at Haridwar station, taking a train to Delhi. The station was bustling and noisy, but he saw a young woman sleeping on the platform with a baby beside her, undisturbed by the commotion. She had covered her face with her saree pallu to keep the flies away. One hand was bent over her forehead, the other hand she placed on her infant's tummy. After a while her baby woke up and moved; the woman turned towards the baby's side, pallu still covering her face, eyes still closed.

The baby got on all fours and crawled a bit. His mother didn't move. Emboldened, he took some more steps away from her. Then, with eyes still closed, she stretched out her hand and pulled the baby back. This happened a couple of times, and soon enough the baby learnt where he could crawl out to without risking being pulled back.

This woman, Swamiji said, should be your meditation teacher. Not some old, saffron-clad, bearded man, he added, referring to himself. Learning to do your duties without being disturbed by the commotion outside, letting your thoughts know where they can go and pulling them back every time they wandered beyond the *seema*, the boundary – this was meditation.

Meditation is for everyone, whether you are a young mother, a coder, a householder, a mathematician. It is an inner state. It's about forgetting that you have a child and taking a nap, but not letting the child forget that it has a parent. It's about not forgetting your true essence, your *astitva*, your true being. Meditation is about being at ease.

It's a lesson I feel is valid for health, too. It's about being at ease with the body, or being in the state where you forget about the body. And yet the body knows that it will get pulled back if it does wander. It's about being at ease with the changes it goes through, the food we eat, the life we lead. It's less about the displays outside, whether it's counting steps in the day or our heart rate in the night, and more about not losing *din ka chain* and *raat ki neend*. Our life will have its ups and downs, but there is no need to lose that sense of ease with oneself. '*Babumoshai, zindagi badi honi chahiye, lambi nahi,*' said Rajesh Khanna to Amitabh Bachchan in the movie *Anand*.

In a *badi zindagi*, it's about knowing that if one's weight, HbA1c, BP or cholesterol climbs a bit, then before running after the numbers you do the first things first. Turn to your side and stretch your hand to pull them back. A healthy person knows that you can forget the numbers, but they should not forget that you are watching them.

So, what does this mean in real life? It's about being less conflicted about food choices, to begin with. Eating correctly is pretty commonsensical and not half as complicated as it's made out to be. Before people try the basics – eating more at home, ordering less from outside, making exercise a part of life, sleeping on time – they download apps, programs and hire professionals who run them out of the money, confidence and bandwidth needed to lead a normal life.

We seem to have forgotten that between doing nothing and chasing weight loss or health as a life goal, there lies a state where just being aware or watchful about food, exercise and sleep could reap excellent results. That's the state where you can watch over the child, nap, stop flies from sitting on your face and still not miss the train. A state where you could literally do it all, optimally. Because an optimum life is one where health and happiness is default and not goals to be chased.

> ### Happy weight
>
> Post three babies, my editor, now in her late forties, said to me that she only follows what I say (credit *toh mein bohot logo ke* good shape and good looks *ka khati hu*). So she lost all her weight after the baby. 'Very good, Chiki,' I said to her, 'And you look fab.'
>
> 'Thanks, but now I am 60 kg. You know, all my life I have been 54 kg but now I don't stress about it. I call this my happy weight. The weight I keep while I exercise, eat all my food, have a drink here and there, and manage work and kids.'
>
> 'Chiki, our bodies change, there's no such thing as "all my life",' I told her. 'This is life too. With two kids, one husband, one start-up, staff, work, an office to look after, yoga to do, authors to chase, deals to crack – for all you know 54 kg was just your "happy weight" for the last decade. If you had been strict then, maybe you would have been 48 kg at the time. But then you would have been so uptight and stressed about keeping that weight that you wouldn't have built half the life you have now.'

> The thing is that at 58 kg or 53 kg (or 65 or 60, 85 or 82), we look pretty much the same – in good shape, and even fit. There is nothing to be achieved by going 5 kg under at all costs. But there is a lot to lose – sanity, focus and, most importantly, joy. So, the realization that the happy weight shifts every decade has to come. But even for that, you must eat right.

Transformations

Radhika came to my office all dressed up. 'I want a selfie with you,' she told me when I entered the room. Only thirty-five, she had been dieting since she was fifteen. 'Two times I have done drastic transformation, once for my wedding (at nineteen), 85 to 50 kilos, and then after childbirth (at twenty-five), from 90 to under 60 kilos.' She had been to eight famous dietitians and ten not-so-famous ones. 'I have given good results to everyone,' she told me proudly. *Kabhi khud pe, kabhi halat pe rona aaya*, was playing in my mind, and then she broke down.

Sniffling, she said to me, 'I didn't want to look like this, pointing to her running kajal. I want to look good in the selfie.'

'You will,' I assured her, 'meeting *ke baad mein lete hain* photo.'

Then she cried through the whole meeting, poor thing. 'When I look back at my pics, I wonder why I was thinking that I am fat,' she said mournfully. (If I had a rupee for every time I have heard this, I would beat the Ambanis at net worth). Calorie counting, step counting, low fat, low carb, detox, fasting, panchakarma, juicing, Ayurvedic cleanses and clinics, and at least eight celeb dietitians later, her weight was now in the triple digits.

And here she was, hoping for another transformation – she had signed up for my three-month program. '*Abhi body ko nahi, attitude ko transform karenge*,' I told her. '*Apne ko* approach *naya lena padega*. This time you do it slowly, sustainably. *Jo baat sui se ho sakti hai, wahan talwar nahin vaprenge*.'

Radhika had listed three program outcomes for herself: 1. Drastic transformation, 2. Don't like being fat, want to get thin, and 3. Get rid of my health problems and have good skin.

But what she was really looking for was something totally different. It was love, acceptance, approval. What was missing in her and in many people I work with isn't discipline, will power or consistency, but an inability to pursue fulfilment, meaning and purpose. Constantly being in the loop of dieting takes us far away from finding that real connect, purpose and joy in life. And no amount of weight loss or transformation can substitute for the real thing. The real thing is to have the fuel to live a full life. Train, baccha, nap, *sab kuchh*.

On science, statistics and stories

Science has made tremendous progress in understanding and describing how our world works, including how we work. But any scientist worth their salt will summarize our current knowledge of the human body[1] as follows: 'We know a lot more than before, but there is so much more yet to know.' From our brain to our gut to our hormones and immune system, there is so much we don't understand fully. But we are making progress every day, and surely in our lifetime we will know ourselves a lot better.

Especially in the field of nutrition, and health in general, where our current best research methods are just not adequate to account for the complex interactions and effects of the environment, pollution, stress, exercise, genes, hormones, neurotransmitters, gut microbiome, etc., on our body, our health and our well-being. The reductionist approach, of breaking down food to its basic molecules and studying them in isolation, has left us with huge gaps in our understanding of food and its relationship with health.

The randomized control trials (RCTs) and the associated statistics are the gold standard in drug trials, where it allows us to tease out the impact of a single ingredient/medicinal compound vis-à-vis a placebo. But in nutrition science, it is extremely difficult to design and implement an RCT due to many inherent and practical factors.[2]

Most of the studies are therefore observational, and although we have collected huge amounts of data, the problems of selective reporting and over-interpreting a single study out of context, and so on, have led to more confusion than clarity. Not to mention the very important statistical and scientific measure of reproducibility,[3] i.e., the need for scientific claims to be replicated by independent researchers, which is, to say the least, missing big time. Combine that with the high degree of interference by the food and weight-loss industries in basic research, and we are on a very sticky wicket.

In the absence of clarity from research and data, we tend to rely more on stories, and once we are in that realm, the story that you hear most often wins, regardless of how scientifically and statistically sound it is. Just like you can design your study in a way that certain outcomes are guaranteed, you can tell the story that best suits your interests. And if you are the food industry, that interest is profits. Social media, with its confident influencers and slick reels, plays a big role in ensuring we hear that story loud and clear, and repeatedly.

So, what's our best bet? Science, statistics and stories, again. A fundamental way in which science progresses is through trial and error, and that's exactly how ancient cultures have fine-tuned their cuisine and crop cycles, ensuring that they get the best nutrition from the available resources and made steady progress in their health outcomes. Our ancestors have done all the hard work and left us with their wisdom, not in the form of research papers, yes, but as recipes, food combinations, rules, and so on – a different format but by no means lacking in scientific rigour.

They have also helped resolve some of the biggest limitations in statistics – the size of the sample set and the duration of the study – by conducting their trials at the population level, over centuries, in real-world living conditions (instead of 'under lab conditions'). And all this science and statistics reaches us in the form of oral wisdom – as stories, songs and proverbs on food and living that our grandmothers tell us gently, in a language of love. Across the globe, across all native cultures, this wisdom has one thing in common – it has the hallmark of **common sense,** and when it comes to food, nutrition and health, it is the **gold standard** to aspire for.

This book

And that's why this book. It has three sections: Diets, *Ghar Ka Khaana* and Commonsense Eating and Living. I wanted to keep the focus on two things: 1. Avoiding dieting and instead eating *ghar ka khaana* is not just commonsense, it is also what the latest in nutrition science is advocating, and 2. Following some commonsense guidelines and rules of *ghar ka khaana,* you can gain health, lose weight and save yourself the time and stress that modern dieting brings, thereby utilizing your bandwidth for the more meaningful pursuits in life.

I have liberally used real conversations with my clients as a means to emphasize a point, and in a language that is relatable. In fact, as much as possible, I have avoided technical jargon as I feel what we all are looking for is *seedhi baat, no bakwaas*. In addition to real examples, there are, as always, boxes – for emphasis, anecdotes, additions – to the main text of the chapters. Last but not the least, there are real diet recalls, along with modifications, to kind of put all the learnings in clear 'what to do' terms.

But underneath these practical sections run some bigger questions: What does it mean to be healthy? What role does food play? What is a full life? I wrote this book so that you don't short-change yourself into just getting thin or losing weight, or looking at forty how you did at twenty and somehow think that this makes up for living a full life. Our aim as humans is to change, to grow, to adapt and to even die, but with fuel in the tank so that it is a worthy ride. If my first book was about size zero, then this one is about living one hundred per cent. It's about gaining health and not about losing weight. Will you lose weight while at it? Yes. But it will also give you the zest and solace of having lived fully, wholly, freely.

Happy reading!

Rujuta Diwekar
Mumbai

Section 1

Diets Don't Work

Carbs

Keto

Spices

Protein

Calories

DIETS DON'T WORK

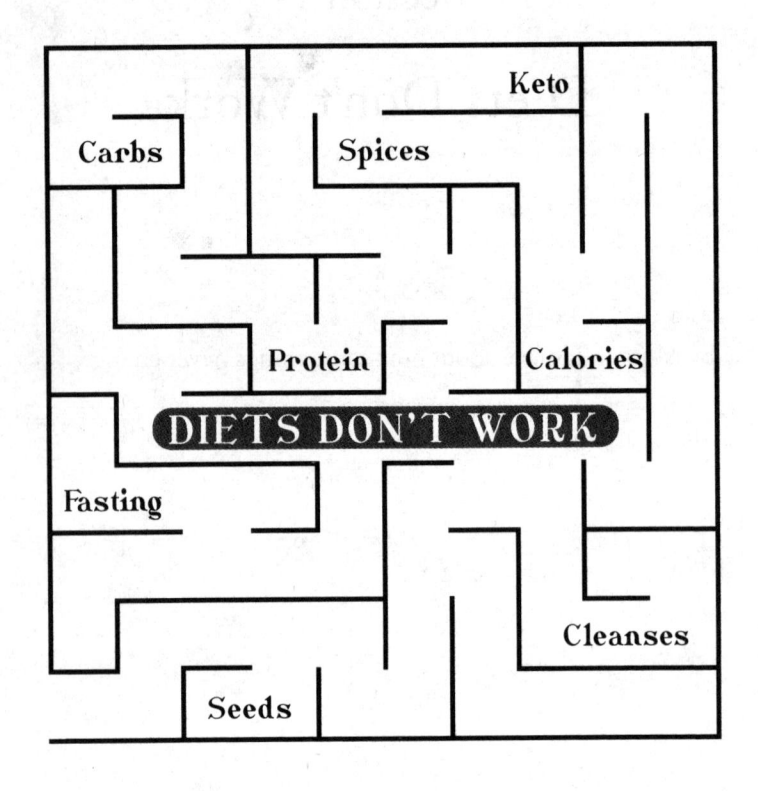

Fasting

Cleanses

Seeds

Same old diets

They say that the more things change, the more they remain the same. *Same as Ever* also happens to be the latest hit book by Morgan Housel about how some things never change, no matter what. I especially love Housel's story of the legendary marathon runner Eliud Kipchoge, because my team and I had heard him speak at a sports conference in Newcastle in 2014 and loved his low-key, confident vibe.

In his book, Housel talks about how, after winning the marathon in the Tokyo Olympics, Kipchoge was sitting in a staging room with the silver and bronze winners, waiting to receive his medal. The three men had to sit in that cramped room for many hours before the ceremony. The two other runners spent their time on their phones while Eluid sat there calmly the entire time, staring at the wall in front of him, as if taking all of it in.

Housel observed that extra-human performances come always from people who don't seem human, who are a little distanced from human emotions that one would typically experience. And how this quality runs through most of the world's super achievers no matter what they have done and when.

There is something similar going on in the dieting world as well. Regardless of what the diet is and when it was introduced, the feature that runs through all of them is deprivation. And even when the old diets come back with new names, the deprivation stays. So, Atkins is keto, low calorie is low carb, skipping dinner is now skipping breakfast/ intermittent fasting, and not eating anything at all is cleanse/ detox. *Naam bade, darshan chhote*. Dirtier, nastier, noisier. Dieting is now a 'lifestyle'. People are on all sorts of lifestyles, and everything is getting cultish and sensitive. You may say anything about their mother but not about their diets.

If you have lived in Mumbai, you have seen it go from Bombay to Mumbai, Elphinstone Road to Prabhadevi. While I am all for reclaiming heritage and using the vernacular, this still hurts. It hurts because other than changing the name, the self-serving politicians aspire to change nothing else. We remain subjects and not citizens. Our cities are still poorly planned, the garbage is still piling, the civic problems still exist and, in fact, have exponentially increased. So what does this name change achieve?

Now, if you bring mass mobility, walkability, green cover and maidans to the city, then you achieve health for many versus profits for a few. That's how you write your name on our hearts instead of plastering your face on hoardings. *Aur waise bhi*, a rose is still a rose, *koi bhi naam se pukaro*. Diets are exactly like that – postured as better because of the change in their names, but still leaving your wallet thin, not your waist.

'Sciency'

So, what's new in 2025? This time, the same old diets and the underlying deprivation are dressed up in 'science' – a lot of it. Food, or eating right, is no longer wholesome or nurturing, it is 'scientific'. I like the term 'sciency' better. Because that's all that it really is.

Science, actually, is pretty simple. Like love, it is repeatable and reproducible. Prashant Damle, a celebrated Marathi stage actor, has a beautiful couplet which sends his audience wild – *'Prem mhanje prem mhanje prem asta, tumcha aani aamcha, ekdum same asta.'* ('Love is love. Whether it's yours or ours, it's exactly the same.') It's *sadak chhaap* for the principles of repeatability and reproducibility. When you love, you have feelings of warmth and tenderness for that person over and over again, to the end of time.

'Through thick and thin, health and sickness' is not a vow we make only when we get married. When there's love, this becomes default. Reproducibility means that when others are in love, their lives are uplifted, just like yours, with the same experience of warmth and tenderness. In science, repeating an experiment over and over is an important step to check that your result is not a matter of chance but actual facts.

Let's say you think cutting back on starch or carbs is crucial, so you quit rice. If you have a scientific bent of mind, you must check if it gets you to lose weight every time. Mostly, it will be: 'It worked for me at twenty-five, but at twenty-seven it's not working,' so it's not repeatable. And reproducibility would mean that all non-rice eaters would be, by default, thin, but we know that people in rice-dominant cultures, be it in Himachal or Northeast India, are not fat. You can replace rice with anything that you believe is 'scientific' at the moment – intermittent fasting, spice shots, cleanses – and you will have different results with the same person every time.

So the basic test of scientific rigour is not fulfilled. Anything that is not repeatable and reproducible is 'sciency', a random occurrence due to conditions not fully accounted for or understood. Just because some self-appointed guardian on X or influencer on Insta or an article on the front page of a newspaper shouts it out or a video on it goes viral, it doesn't become solid science. It remains just that – sciency.

To make matters more complicated, now there is also the dressing of culture. If nutrition science is saying eat local, as per time-tested traditions, the nutrition industry is all geared up to monetize that too. It has responded by picking up single ingredients from ancient cultures (turmeric, for example) and turning them into miracle foods, and appropriating ancient practices like fasting into weight-loss fads.

Closer home, you can see the market for 'herbal', '*satvik*' products booming along with practices like consuming seeds and spices as shots, doing gut cleanses, and the like. 'But it is part of our ancient tradition' is now added to the 'but this is scientific' argument. It is now hard to tell the pseudo-science from the pseudo-cultural.

The pursuit of the futile

They say there is no such thing as an original thought or idea. Everything that you can think about or write about has already been thought and written about. Long before *Same as Ever* highlighted how the same things are at work, Sage Patanjali, in his seminal work, *The Yoga Sutras*, expounded on the *kleshas* (faults) that keep us engaged in the futile. *Raga, dvesha, abhinivesha* exist within each one of us, and can be used to manipulate us into doing unreasonable things. You will see that with the dieting world too.

Raga is loosely translated as 'attachment'. The attachment to your body can be used to get you on a diet that will make you look even more attractive or thinner. Reminds me of a client of mine who went on a diet when she was 56 kg to look thinner for her engagement. She was twenty-four at the time. When we next met, she was forty-two, and she said, 'Looking back, I wonder what was I even thinking, because today, even if I get under 80 kg, I will dance with joy.'

Dvesha translates to a kind of hatred. Hating the way one looks is also used to put people on a diet, and then you are automatically off all the food that provides you comfort. So no more rice for you, only protein, and if you can't poop, get some fibre or laxatives. It's not good enough that you hate the way you look, you must also hate all that you eat.

Abhinivesha, the will to live long or not die. 'Don't eat sugar, it is killing you.' So going off fresh fruit or drinking *feeki chai*, or fasting for long hours to extend your life, etc.

The wellness and weight-loss industry has always deployed *raga*, *dvesha* and *abhinivesha* to their benefit, but today it is amplified by social media. And the industry is booming like never before. Where once it had school dropouts or low scorers (like me) struggling to make a living, it is now awash with funding, attracting the IIT, IIM, Ivy League types, who want last-mile connectivity for diets. Coach, Dt., are the new titles. And doctors – from gynaecologists to cardiologists – are offering food, exercise and relationship advice for visibility and traction.

The lucrative field is now also a second career option for those who are bored with being chartered accountants, media professionals, programmers and the like. *Behti Ganga mein sabko haath dhona hai.* And your next-door neighbour is just three months and one social media account away from being the newest expert in town. Or maybe everyone was always an expert but now they are using good lighting, good angles and algorithms to land on your timeline.

Diets Don't Work

Chhaapkar bikte the joh kabhi,
bik kar chhaapte hain woh abhi

What would once sell after being published is now sold first and then published. Someone said this about *akhbaars* (mainstream newspapers) and when I first heard it, I didn't understand what it meant. They were talking about paid articles coming across as news and the loss of transparency in general. Years have passed, but this *kahawat* has stayed with me. Mostly because I receive emails that read, 'Hi Madam. Below are the media-approved headlines, can you please write an 800-word article on "Ignorance leads to protein deficiency amongst students and working professionals", "Protein myths busted", "Alarming health impacts of protein deficiency", "Your breakfast lacks 80% protein", etc.' The page, the space and the headline are locked first, and the article is written by a 'credible voice' later.

Earlier, this was limited to films or politics, but now the trend has penetrated every sphere of life. And food and fitness are probably the most 'written' about. Social media marketing has made advertorials masked as editorials look lame and harmless in comparison. From ₹1,500 crores in 2023, the social media influencer market in India is set to grow to a whopping ₹3,375 crores in 2026. By 2029, we are expected to be the largest social media market. Influencers will tell you everything you need to know – what to wear, what to eat, what to think. And we will all be consuming advertisements masked as information, science or secrets.

So, in this section, we look at both the 'sciency' diets and the 'pseudo-cultural' trends, and why they don't work.

1

'Sciency' diets

1. Playing with nutrients – high protein/low carb, etc.

'That's it, Rujuta ben, I just couldn't do it anymore,' said Hiral bhai to me, in response to my question – what made him get off his diet. He was a forty-two-year-old insurance broker with a twelve-year-old son, a wife, parents and a booming business to look after. He was always overweight, but after turning forty he had decided, *iss baar NO sau paar*. From 112 kg he had dropped to 96 kg in less than two months, but now it had become challenging to keep up with the diet. His target was 75 kg, but he couldn't bear the thought of following his diet for even one more day!

'*Kya diet hai aap ka?*' I asked. Fifty-two cubes of cheese a week and 1 kg of paneer! With that he was allowed some boiled veggies and one bowl of sprouts a day. Boiled veggies *mein bhi* only broccoli and bhindi, no aloo or *kacha kela*, and *agar rice khane ka man hua* (only if he was really lacking in will power), he was allowed 'rice' made out of cauliflower. And his treat was an almond-flour khakra filled with seeds, or a flourless chocolate cake. '*Mohanthal wala cake kaisa khayega? Term cover wale ko money-back chipka diya.* Only agent is making money. *Waise* my dietitian is now saying constipation *hai toh fibre supplement lo. Neend nahi aati hai toh magnesium supplement lo.*'

You talk to the guy, he's smart. He says his business has solid potential. Most of India is not insured and he plans to change that. 'But insurance,' he said, '*dil aur trust ka mamla hai. Kya hai, bure waqt mein agent ne dhoka diya toh business khallas.*' He said from fire to house to medical to car to accident claims, *kitna bhi magaj lage*, he ensures that his client gets the money. Especially in case of an untimely death. The family must not suffer.

'Hiral bhai,' I said, '*yeh cheese cubes, paneer meals and cauli rice banake bhi family suffer hi hota hai. Marne ki zaroorat hi nahi hai.*'

'That's right,' he said. 'My wife is saying that *tere ko abhi na neend aati hai, na potty, sirf gussa aata hai.*'

The thing with diets getting nastier is that people on them are getting angrier. Having been in this profession all my adult life, I can tell you one thing for sure – being 'hangry' is real. People are still hungry even if they are now 'allowed' the foods that used to be on the 'strictly avoid' list, like cheese and paneer. I mean, on paper, adding fat to the diet adds satiety, regulates appetite and reduces cravings, but if this comes with no roti, rice or just plain, regular meals, then it's nothing short of a nightmare.

It's one thing to eat fifty-two cubes of cheese over a year, quite another to eat them all in just one week. Somewhere in the 'they got it all wrong, you should have been eating fat all along' we forget that we are *still* getting it wrong. I mean, my *thakela* joke is that *pehle dukhi log pav bhaji mein butter avoid karte the, ab woh pav avoid karte hai.*

> ## Carb fear
> the irrational belief that eating home-cooked meals like roti-sabzi, dal-chawal, poha, upma, idli, dosa, thepla, etc., makes one fat or sick, or that they are inadequate in nutrition.

Even if one is not as extreme as Hiral bhai, there is at least some version of carb fear and protein scarcity that everyone feels. Today, a high-protein diet is regarded not just as *the* way to lose weight but also to 'reverse' diseases, no matter how sick you feel doing it. The popular idea nowadays for weight loss is to reduce carbs and increase protein intake. This builds on the general perception that we are all taking in too many carbs and too little protein.

Carb fear among athletes

Every year, me and my team try to attend at least one major international conference on nutrition and/or exercise to keep ourselves up to date with the latest in science and also to present findings from the public health projects we regularly undertake. In December 2022, at the International Sports and Exercise Nutrition conference (ISENC) in Manchester, UK, a session highlighted the carb fear among athletes. The professor spoke about how ageing and most troubles that it brings were to do with loss of muscle strength. And while losing muscle strength with age was inevitable, exercise and protein were good interventions to both preserve and slow down the rate of loss. But the key, the speaker had said, was to have a lot of muscle to begin with. So, while exercise in old age mattered, what mattered even more was the level of activity and athleticism as an adolescent. Exercise worked optimally when the elderly were active adolescents. That way, they had a muscle bank to draw from, a neuromuscular pathway that just needed some brushing up, etc. And this was useful even if they were not very active in their middle age.

Similarly, the other intervention of protein worked optimally when there was no carb fear. The speaker went on to define carb fear as an irrational fear of eating regular foods like fruits, nuts, grains, legumes, etc. When protein was consumed at the cost of wholesome food, it didn't work like the way it was meant to – adding muscle size and strength.

> Instead, it took away from the gains that could be made. And as human life extends, diseases are going to come to everyone's homes, so the conversation is going to shift to health outcomes. If two people of the same age get the same disease (her research was on the size of tumours), then the chances of death, recurrences and complications were reduced for those with better muscle strength.

Kirti's misfortune

The eat-more-protein-and-cut-carbs bug has bitten everybody. My mom is a little over seventy, a retired organic chemistry teacher whose friends are all high and mighty in intellect. One afternoon, they were having a get-together at their friend, Pratibha's. The grey hair and grey cells were going to share a good meal and a good laugh. Some of them had lost their partners to death and their children to foreign soil. But they hadn't lost their spirit or the will for debate, gossip and food. But then my mom's confidante, Kirti, called and said, 'Rekha, I can't come.' 'Why?' my mother demanded. 'Listen, I must eat 45 grams of protein for lunch and I can't ask Pratibha to do that.'

My mother's bff had done her blood tests and her HbA1c was 5.9. She had been advised to lose weight. Her weight is 57 kg. She is seventy-four years old, is driven and committed in all aspects of her life, so she was going to fix this. Naturally.

Her doctor had put her on a 'protein-rich' diet – no sugar, no carbs, a green smoothie daily or 100 g of boiled greens at every meal.

She was game for it, anything to avoid having her kids let go of their lives and take care of her in her old age, even if it meant avoiding gup-shup with the girl gang she had been friends with for half a century.

'No way,' my mother said. She called Pratibha, and Pratibha called Kirti. 'Kirti, you must come, don't worry about me. *Mein laga degi cooker mein tere liye 45 g of chhole. Khali seeti hi toh marna hai.* You come.' So Kirti came and ate only the boiled chhole.

My mother had brought tomato saar. 'Have this,' she said to her, 'instead of the green smoothie.'

'But Rekha, this has sugar, right?'

'But only 1 tsp between six of us and six tomatoes.'

Another friend had gotten vangi kaap, tava-roasted aubergine that uses rava and rice flour, but she lied to Kirti and said, 'I didn't put rice flour because Pratibha called me and said that you are avoiding rice.'

I think the way to reverse diseases naturally is to invest in a girl gang. They don't judge you when you go off-track and always bring you back into the fold. They always let you be, they scold you a bit, they lie to you a bit, but they let you be. And honestly, sometimes that's all you need.

Kirti was a quintessentially disciplined Tam Bram. She cooked all her meals at home, led a regulated life and always had her weight in check. She did three days of yoga a week and had continued online even during the pandemic. That's how her lipid profile was good, her triglycerides well under 150 and her thyroid was healthy. But *saala* HbA1c was out of range, so *baat khatam*. This test result had come post-pandemic, when she was seventy-four years old. Her medical advice should have used context – the anxiety of the lockdown, kids abroad, etc.

A woman who ate everything at home, prayed, invested four to five hours in yoga every week and got to seventy-five without a single disease should be spared of radical advice, an unrealistic diet in this case. Her routine, in fact, should be studied. She should be appreciated for looking after herself so well. At the most she could be asked to add a day of strength training every week, resume regular activities and repeat the test after three months.

Carbs are not the bad boy

Eliminating carbs is not the magic pill it's made out to be and doesn't work, just like eliminating fat didn't work years ago.

1. People who advise you to cut down carbs and increase fibre for weight loss, diabetes, etc., are contradicting themselves in the same breath. Grains, millets, legumes are excellent sources of fibre, and not just fruits or green leafy vegetables.
2. Avoiding carbs – paratha, dosa, bhakri, roti, rice, poha, upma, and so on – deprives the body of wholesome

> nutrition, and leads to palate and bodily fatigue. Aches, pains, poor sleep and digestion, etc.
> 3. Without carbs, the brain experiences loss of fuel, decision-making becomes difficult, and there is confusion – 'brain fog' – irritability and anxiety.

Kirti followed her diet diligently, became a gaunt 49 kg from 57 kg and lowered her HbA1c to 5.6. But soon enough, signs of weakness began to show. She now needed her maid to help her into her blouse. Her shoulders hurt. She began to avoid backbends in yoga because her back and knees would hurt. She started getting restless legs and sleepless nights. Her digestion got poorer. But she attributed all that to her age and not to the changes she had made in her diet. An aviyal–sambar–sundal person was now a 45 g-protein, 100 g-green veggies, zero-sugar person. It was bound to go wrong.

Good health isn't just about HbA1c or any one parameter. It is also about standing on our two feet, laughing with our friends, sharing our meals, exchanging recipes, doing a smooth Ustrasana in a yoga class that erupts into a spontaneous applause. I mean, at seventy-five you are on borrowed time that much more than what you are when you are forty-five or thirty-five, so you must make the most of it, no?

But is there really a protein gap?

> **Protein gap**
> The misplaced notion that most populations, especially vegetarians, are deficient in protein.

The 'Politics of Protein' report by the International Panel of Experts on Sustainable Food Systems (IPES-Food) has conclusively shown that there is no such thing as a 'global protein gap'. The only people who fall short on protein are the ones who fall below the poverty line, and this is because they do not have access to adequate food – at least no access to adequate nutritious food on all days. Now just turn that around. People simply need access to nutritious, real food to get their protein or the in-vogue nutrient of the decade.

Nor should you need to worry about protein insufficiency because you are a vegetarian. In India, a lot of those who suffer from poverty are likely to be meat eaters. And yet they fall short on protein. Because nutrient deficiencies, including those of protein, are not about whether you are a vegetarian, eggetarian, non-vegetarian, pescan, vegan, etc. – it's about whether you are poor.

I can safely say that if you bought and are reading this book, you are not poor. It's like the cliché: In the world that counts its carbs, calories and steps, be a rebel and count your blessings. If your plate is full, your protein intake is adequate. If you really care about protein, support the government when it gets into welfare mode and wants to bring access to nutritious food for everyone.

And if you do want to be vigilant about your protein intake, then care about getting a diverse range of proteins on your plate – dals and legumes, nuts, dairy-based protein like milk and dahi, and fish, meat and eggs if you are a non-vegetarian.

In summary, *a shortage of protein doesn't exist, and surely doesn't exist in isolation.* The ones who are falling short of it are falling short of all nutritious things, including access to education, sanitation, dignity and income. So, removing carbs and consuming protein tries to fix what is not broken.

The politics of protein[4]

Released in April 2022, this is the most comprehensive report on protein till date, put together by the International Panel of Experts on Sustainable Food Systems (IPES-Food). They look at the bigger picture of why there is such a hype for protein and point out the concentration of the meat and dairy business in a handful of companies globally (called 'big protein', who, incidentally, also have big investments in alternative protein start-ups). The report says that the exploding market for protein products is also driving the narrative of protein insufficiency. The panel's recommendation is simple but far reaching: There is no global protein gap except when people struggle with poverty,

> and instead of a protein transition, we should drive a global transition towards sustainable food systems, a.k.a. local, seasonal and traditional.
>
> You can read more at www.ipes-food.org

Protein – consumption vs assimilation

The key to protein assimilation is its digestibility. Consuming protein, its assimilation, and then the sparing of protein for growth, repair and maintenance are not quite the same thing. Currently, the narrative is entirely focused on consumption. And from weight loss to disease prevention, from good skin to longevity – it is the answer to everything. The reality, though, is very different.

When people get protein-consumption focused, they miss out on rice, poha, chapati, bhakri, to start with. Then, of course, they also miss out on fresh fruit – banana, mango, sitaphal *ka toh naam bhi lena allowed nahi hai*. And then, from pumpkin seeds to pistachios, everything is eaten just for protein. So it's chia seeds in the morning; eggs, avocado and cheese for breakfast; grilled chicken with salad or sautéed veggies for lunch; a protein shake thrown in; and meat, fish, egg or paneer for dinner. You expect to feel fab but you fart, unexpectedly. But don't worry, there's a cure for that too: fibre drinks, pills and powders.

And how can I forget the probiotic yogurt? The more unpronounceable the brand, the better it works. Every actor, cricketer and creator worth their salt is now into products that are ready-to-eat and sell you health. Good business sense is about having a fat bottom line, and what better way to do it than to pitch it on a slim waist line? See, I have told you this, but I will tell you again: What's good for profits is often bad for people and the planet. In the nineties, actors and cricketers would squander their money, now they triple it with investments in food companies and do the ads for free.

And nothing wrong with that. I for one love money and so I am careful where I put it. So should you. Any weight loss (even if it comes) that comes at the cost of not eating simple, sensible *ghar ka khaana* is going to eat away at that muscle tissue that you are trying so hard to preserve. And losing muscle is never going to make you look thinner, only flabbier. And disproportionate, too. And no, exercise is not going to save or help you build more muscle if you are restricting home-cooked food and the seasonal staples of fruits and veggies.

All that exercise will do then is cause exertion and injuries, not to mention gastric distress. And instead of figuring out where you are going wrong by watching what you eat, you are going to watch the internet and diagnose that your low energy and frequent injuries are being caused by low protein, so you are going to add some more to your diet. And then that consumption–exertion–injury–distress cycle is going to go on till frustration hits (because it always does), and then you are going to eat cake, cheat with a biryani or worse, get a pizza or pancakes.

Then you are going to feel guilty and go into repeat mode till your body finally not just refuses to budge on the weight but also seeks revenge by going up on body weight and HbA1c, breaking out into acne, etc. So, now you must smarten up and eat 'smart carbs', the friend, guide and philosopher will tell you. 'What's "smart carbs"?' I asked a client who was telling me this story. 'Oh, it's dals, legumes, grapefruit.' Then, over time, this too will not get you what you want but just ABC – acidity, bloating, constipation – and you will finally hang up your high-protein boots. Or at least that's my hope.

> ## The food matrix
> It refers to a food's physical structure, the way the molecules inside it interact, and how this interplay affects the way we digest and absorb nutrients.

When we eat food like it is available in nature, without tinkering with its nutrients, we stand to gain the most out of the goodness it offers. For example, the assimilation of protein from whole milk is better than low-fat milk, including low-fat milk with added amino acids. The lesser the processing, the better the access to nutrients.

Same with whole egg – it offers more nourishment than the whites of two eggs. And in the greed to get more protein and keeping the fat intake down, eating six egg whites really offers no benefit as compared to eating two eggs with toast, like the way you naturally would if you could put the protein mania aside.

Even post-workout protein assimilation to aid recovery peaks when protein comes with a combination of carbs. So, have that banana with your protein shake or have a paneer paratha or egg curry with rice. It would be better any day than just a protein shake post-workout.

Essentially, the food matrix just tells us what we already know – it's the full package and not the single nutrient that matters. The package of other essential nutrients, wholesome taste and ease of digestion is crucial in order to meet the body's protein requirements. You often use the word 'package' when talking about a job, you even use it to describe a great guy because a great guy is more than just good looks and a package is more than just salary.

'Horses for courses,' Ravi Shastri, arguably India's most successful coach, would have said. Every player who's made it to the squad is good, but some are better for certain pitches. Your body is a bit like that. If you just eat protein at the cost of not eating carbs or home-cooked food, it simply breaks down protein and uses it for energy purposes – basically it will use the molecule for all non-exclusive protein work too. Now that's just a waste of time, digestive enzymes and money. Also, protein doesn't have wings, so eat excess of it and it gets converted to fat, just like eating excess cake does. *Toh problem kya hai? Excess ka.* Once you get that, you get everything right in life.

Exercise and sleep

Alongside digestibility, we must consider two other critical aspects – exercise and sleep. Both are underrated but crucial for the assimilation of protein.

Exercise leads to the calibrated wear and tear of our muscle tissue, and the body needs this dose of breakdown to stimulate muscle protein synthesis (i.e., to build muscle). Consistency with exercise is the most crucial aspect of the assimilation of protein. Aim for a minimum dose of 150 minutes a week.

Sleep – without it, any amount of exercise or protein intake is pretty much useless. Sleep is when most, if not all, the repair work takes place.[5] If you are eating protein for better hormone production – growth hormone, insulin, testosterone, etc. – sleep becomes even more critical for you. Men need about seven to eight hours of sleep a day, and women can need up to nine hours around hormonal milestones.

What about protein shakes?

Yes, a protein shake is fine, but the problem often is that the protein shake, in the absence of a wholesome diet, is just not effective. And exercise will then only lead to exhaustion, injuries and frequent illnesses. You can just skip the protein shake if it doesn't sit well in your stomach and have a wholesome meal instead (within thirty minutes of working out).

Context matters the most

I have many problems with the protein narrative, but easily the biggest one is that it is far removed from our cultural context. Context *kya hai bhai*? The United States Department of Agriculture (USDA), in its latest dietary guidelines, lays emphasis on healthy diets as those diets that are formulated according to personal preferences, cultural traditions and are within budgetary means. That is what context means. Kirti's is a case in point, but hers isn't the only one.

I recently came across a tweet from a health influencer who routinely warns people not to believe advice on social media, sharing his advice for how vegetarians should get their protein, especially if they are pregnant.

Against every item, he had written the grams of protein. I will spare you the details, but I will tell you the list. It started with Greek yoghurt, went on to peanut butter, quinoa and pumpkin seeds, and ended with tempeh, edamame, etc. I mean, *aaj tak apni aabadi bina yeh kuchh khaye kaise badh rahi hai*? But jokes apart, imagine a pregnant girl who is barely able to tolerate the sight, smell and thought of food, who is trying to get a grip on her digestion and struggling to sleep, trying to ingest these? Yes, food tweets bring better traction, but do you notice the lack of home-food options on that list?

And where does the truth really lie? That dry fruit that your mother, aunt, mother-in-law or older friend goads you to eat; the ragi or besan laddoo that your neighbour lovingly sends; the sensitivity that your friends show in not smoking in front of you or going out for dinner early now that you are pregnant, are all that one needs. A few extra calories (nutritious, of course, *chadho mat mere pe*) and a little TLC make all the difference.

The lawyer who was made of steel

A client of mine was a successful lawyer – a partner at her firm. Not too many women last that long. But she was made of steel, of nerves, wit and diligence. Every year she would do a routine blood test. No one had ordered them, it was just diligence on her part. Her numbers were all in range, and all the t's had been crossed and i's dotted.

Then, for a year after she turned forty, she went on the usual protein diet. She ate more protein than ever and lifted weights. This time she expected to see even better reports, but to her dismay that was not the case.

She told Jinal from my team that she had come with one agenda – to figure out what was going wrong with her. She had a job, a little son, an ailing mother, a husband with a fancy job, a trainer, a Vedanta class, volunteering work at a blind school (part-time two days a month). She had a cook, a nanny and a nurse, but things weren't right. 'I am crashing, or at least that is how I feel. I always do an annual blood report, and that's when I saw that my protein levels were really low.'

'When my doctor saw it, he said look, this explains the constant low energy. Just eat more protein. But if I do that, then I have to just quit my job and eat protein full time. Because just look at my eating sheet (referring to her three-day diet recall). I only eat protein. I am already eating 120 g, do I up it to 150–170 g?' That's also how she had lost weight. But the main thing was that she felt tired. Very tired. All the time. And she was tired of feeling tired.

'Have you also cut out all carbs?' Jinal asked.

'Obviously,' she replied.

'Ok, let's add them back.'

So, we had her eat a toast with her two eggs. Which kind of toast? 'Anything you prefer,' said Jinal. We asked her to add rice with her dal. What kind of rice? 'Anything you prefer.' Add a sabzi too. Any one that's fresh from the local sabzi walla. We scaled back on the shakes, just kept the post-workout one and then added a ragi laddoo for an evening snack (handy and quick, can be eaten in a rick or taxi) and post-workout, roti–sabzi or rice–chicken for dinner, and also added a glass of milk before bedtime.

And the report, energy and mood improved. She was happy that her son picked up the ragi laddoo habit and her mother that of haldi milk at night. 'But most importantly,' she told Jinal, 'I no longer snap at my son and have the patience to listen to my mom tell the same story on repeat. I feel less guilty now. Can eating right do that?'

It's not magic, it's chemistry. Maybe it's biochemistry. Maybe it's nothing but the body's way to survive. When you are mindful of what you eat, being mindful of not consuming excess calories, and then get on the protein bandwagon, you begin to fall short of your daily calories. When that happens, not only do you sub-optimally use the protein you eat (break it down) but your body also begins to waste or break down the muscle tissue that it currently holds. Muscle is an expensive tissue to keep. And if there's going to be a food shortage, the body is trained to get rid of muscle and prioritize survival.

Like all women, my client had to juggle multiple roles and work. So just because she turned forty nothing terrible was going to happen to her. The same old things would continue, but now she had to just be kinder to herself, not go on a punishing diet. So, ya, don't stop that dahi–rice, banana, roti–sabzi – regular home-cooked food, really. Because they are like that soft breeze, tender gaze and mature love that you are missing in your life.

So, how much protein do you really need?

Well, you should know the answer to this by now. Just the routine, home-cooked meals that are diverse, timely, and the ones where you are not overthinking protein, more than get you the grams of protein per kg of body weight that you need. The amount of protein for optimum functioning of the body is quite low, actually, unlike the narrative. Most of the global health organizations and national dietary guidelines, including those of the USA, Canada, the UK, India, etc., recommend a protein intake of between 0.8 g to 1 g per kg of body weight. So for a 60 kg person like me, it's about 48 to 60 g a day.

So if I had breakfast, lunch, dinner and an evening snack and ensured that I am not undereating, I would meet my protein requirements without having to 'up' my protein with a shake or seeds or anything that I am not familiar with. So honestly, we are not short on protein, but we are short on:

- confidence, because we second-guess quantities at every meal and hence fall short on protein.
- vision, because we get protein-focused and stand to lose out on fibre, vitamins, minerals, taste and ease of digestion that regular meals offer.
- adequate exercise and activity, as we spend too much time scrolling on reels that tell us repeatedly that we are falling short of protein and offer expensive solutions like tempeh, tofu, quinoa, etc.
- sleep, again, as we are scrolling reels
- eating home-cooked meals and excessive on junk food, takeout, alcohol and vape – all the stuff that leeches protein out of your body but you won't pay attention to.

So, sorry, but you are short on courage to eat normally. We will discuss this more in detail when we are talking about food combinations and proportions, but for now, here is a quick summary of what not to do to meet your protein requirements:

- Do not need to go out of your traditional practices of food. For example, moving from being a vegetarian to non-vegetarian or eggetarian, etc.

- Do not need to go out of regional practices of food also. For example, inclusion of sattu or makhana. You can do it to share heritage but not as a source of protein.
- Do not need to eat international sources of protein either – edamame or peanut butter or Greek yogurt. When you do, do it for a change, not for protein.
- Do not alter time-tested proportions of food. For example, increasing urad dal in idli prep or moong dal in khichdi.

And a few things to keep in mind

- If you want to switch to being vegan, know that it's much more complicated than the narrative of cruelty or greenhouse gas emissions. It depends on the region of the world you live in, the community/population you belong to, the food systems prevalent in your region, and much more. You must make an informed decision.
- If you are a non-vegetarian, you can continue eating the kind of meat you have traditionally eaten. But follow the time-tested food practices of eating meat a few times a week and as part of a complete meal.
- And finally, at the policy level, the government needs to focus on poverty reduction and food access, and not get distracted by the protein narrative.

> **Devil's advocate**
>
> But what if I am upping my protein more carefully. So instead of two to three rotis and my protein and vegetables, I now eat only one roti and put more protein and vegetables on my plate. Is that a problem?

The one-line answer to this is – you cannot fix what is not broken. You don't need to add any nutrient to your plate carefully, you must just be careful that you are not tinkering the time-tested combinations at the cost of falling short on fibre, magnesium, Vitamin B, and so on. All these are found in grains, millets and legumes; and most 'careful' additions of protein mean deleting these in order to add protein, and then taking supplements to balance all that you carelessly deleted from your food plate.

The thing is that we have made the simple pleasures of life like food extremely complicated. Most often, being on a diet means eating much less than what you would like to because you don't want to consume too many calories. Or it would mean eating in a manner where you are, for example, subtracting the second roti or helping of rice you need, to add an egg or a bowl of paneer or tofu because you want to add more protein.

Or you eat too much of a sabzi or salad in the hope of keeping your overall intake low and your satiety high. You may think that all these are very intelligent strategies, or you may have seen some well-made reels where rice is replaced with some source of protein but what you don't see or know is that nutrition science is now recognizing this phenomenon as **BED – binge-eating disorder.**

Binge-eating disorder is different from the usually diagnosed ones like anorexia or bulimia. But it is an eating disorder, nevertheless. It is an unhealthy obsession with looking a certain way and punishing yourself for not looking hot/reel-worthy/at least 2 kg skinnier. In the age of social media, most girls seem to be on its spectrum (Australia has recently banned social media for teenagers because of the harmful effects it has on their health and confidence). And the tendency is to under-eat at meal times, only to binge late at night or at random times. Net-net, you are not just out of shape but out of self-esteem, too. Instead, sit, chew every bite, engage with food with all your senses, slow down, and repeat the whole exercise. And I promise you that you will not be looking for chocolate, chips or ice cream ever in your life. You may still eat them but only out of a decision and not desperation.

You don't know how liberating that's gonna feel.

2. Playing with calories – intermittent fasting/skipping meals

'Will you talk to my brother? He's one of India's top cardiologists and he cannot believe that I am eating and losing,' my client asked me one day.

'Sure, I will.'

My thumb rule is that the answer to the question 'Will you talk to my brother, mother, sister, wife' is always yes. My clients may have to go through a waiting period before their program starts, but their family will not wait. Family comes first is a rule I like to live by. So, the cardio brother could talk only on a Sunday, and only at 4 p.m., but *'chalega chalega*, no problem'.

'All right, so my sister can't stop talking about you and insisted that I speak to you,' said Dr Sai Satish from the other side. *Bhai koi bhi ho*, they will always act like they are doing their sisters a huge favour.

'Hope good things,' I said, the usual thing to say in these circumstances.

'Oh yeah, but I am already doing IF and I have never felt more energetic, I eat at 2 p.m. and then 8 p.m. So I am going to do this until the end of the year, lose all the weight and then in Jan I will join your program.'

We were talking sometime in October or November. 'Sure, look forward to connecting then,' I said and we hung up.

He called me back the next day.

'Hey, why didn't you say anything to me after I told you that I am doing IF?'

'Nothing,' I said.

'Come on,' he said.

'Seriously, nothing.'

'No, you didn't say what you were thinking. What were you thinking?'

First of all, men don't listen, and if they are doctors they listen even less, and if they are cardiologists, at the top of the chain, they only talk. This one had heard my silence. Bloody impressive. So I opened up and said, 'I was just thinking that if I was ever on your table, I would want my surgery to be scheduled at 4 p.m.' He couldn't stop laughing at the other end.

'Wow, I like you, how soon can we start?'

The sweet middle

The problem in today's world is that we seem to have lost the measure of how much to do. We swing between the extremes of too much and too little, without even once hitting that *Suvarna madhyam*, the sweet middle. Take the case of skipping meals in the hope of eating lesser calories. In the good old times, people skipped dinner. I mean about twenty to twenty-five years ago. That's when I started working and almost everyone I spoke to or worked with, ate soup and salad for dinner because they considered that light. Then they binged in the middle of the night, stayed fat and looked for a dietitian to help them.

That's how I entered the picture. Me saying, 'eat dal–chawal for dinner as a light meal', almost earned me the reputation of being a revolutionary. My clients ate their dal–chawal (I mean, anything to lose weight, ya), didn't feel like bingeing in the night and, lo and behold, lost weight.

Twenty to twenty-five years ago seems like a long time because social media has meant that everything is at a fast forward pace. But the problems of extremes remains unchanged, just as the problem of replacing something good with something poor. If dinner was the villain then, the new villain is breakfast. Now everyone wants to skip breakfast and go straight to lunch at 2 p.m. If dal–chawal was replaced by soup and salad back then, now it's the likes of poha or paratha being replaced by tall black coffees and even a cigarette to go with it.

While there is no doubt that eating packaged cereals, tetra pack juices, jams and spreads is unhealthy, skipping breakfast altogether or just having a coffee instead is a poor deal. I would think this is common sense, but we are living in a world where sciency and spiritualism go hand in hand. Not just the influencer, today even your guru wants you to skip breakfast. Maybe both want you to have your coffee with a shot of ghee. Maybe not. Maybe the doctor is telling you that ghee is trans fat, the guru is telling you it's A2 ghee and cows listen to bhajans daily so it's all good vibes, but all you have now is bad confusion.

The sweet middle here would mean a return to homemade *nashta* instead of packaged cereals. But then, everyone is saying 'skip breakfast/do IF'. Then first check the definition of 'everyone'. Does it translate to health and food influencers with verified handles who land on your timeline? Because everyone is saying other things – your mother is goading you to at least have almonds before leaving home, your daughter is rolling her eyes when you pick up coffee while dropping her off to school and your secretary is now scheduling all your important meetings only after lunch since your temper is flying.

Like mother, like son

A client of mine wanted her fourteen-year-old son to sign up with me.

'Please just check on him, he's terrible with food.'

'Arre, don't worry about him,' I said. 'They are just badly behaved with their mothers but are absolutely ok otherwise.'

'No, no, he's well behaved,' she assured me. 'But *bohot foodie hai.*'

'Oh, don't worry, he will stop making demands,' I said.

'That's the thing,' she clapped her hands in frustration and said. 'He doesn't demand anything. He's fasting. He wakes up and leaves for school without eating anything. On the way to school, he picks up a Starbucks coffee, then he skips the small recess break and only has lunch at 2 p.m. during the big break. But from 11 a.m. to 1.30 p.m., he's unable to focus in class. I even have a calendar note from school.

> 'In the evening, if we are having anything made at home, he won't have it. And we are social people, we have a ton of parties at home but my boy won't touch a thing. *Maa hu mein*,' she said emotionally. 'I know he wants to eat. But he deprives himself, and then come the weekend, there's no stopping his eating and bingeing.'
>
> We have had a generation of forty- to fifty-year-old mommies who have been dieting all through their youth, not knowing that seeking to be thinner at any cost is a contagious disease. When your kids do the nastier, dirtier version of what you did to yourself in your twenties, *toh tum se dekha nahi jaata hai*? When I was growing up, I wanted a better world for women – equality, really. The only place where we have truly achieved it now is that some (not all) boys are as insecure about their looks as young girls.

Knowledge vs information

A doctor recently tweeted that fasting for seventy-two hours kills tumour cells. It went viral, every influencer worth his salt adding their two cents to it – 'The solution to kill cancer is so simple but people lack the "will" or "discipline" to do it.' Or the good old conspiracy theories of how pharma wants to keep you sick for profit or a culture-spin on how ancient cultures have always fasted, etc.

And then Dr Pramesh, who is the director of Tata

Memorial Hospital (TMC Mumbai) and the convenor of National Cancer Grid, which is trying to make cancer care accessible and affordable to all, replied, 'No, it doesn't,' only to receive a healthy dose of backlash.

'What do you know? This person is a doctor, who are you?' asked one user. Dr Pramesh's handle doesn't have a 'doctor' in it; it says @cspramesh. *Username mein doctor nahi, toh tum doctor nahi.*

The thing with knowledge is that the more you know, the less sure you are about what you know and the more you want to learn. And the thing with information is that it gives you the confidence of being well informed, and now you want to teach others.

The fact is that, in India, the incidence of cancer cases are estimated to increase to 2.09 million in 2040 as compared to 1.32 million in 2020, and the number of new patients at Tata Memorial Centres are now 1.28 lakh, an increase of 16 per cent from last year. When you watch all this as a part of your daily life, you know that people are willing to go to any extent to cure themselves, including selling their homes, pulling their children out of school, living on footpaths … all to have access to treatment. And even with proven standard care, which includes multiple interventions like medicines, surgery, etc., the cure or remission rate is dependent on so many factors like age, stage, co-morbidities.

In any case, loss of appetite, aversion to food and nausea are some of the most common side effects of the treatment, and none of them makes you stronger. It just makes it harder for you and for the caregiver, but people brave it. So, if a single intervention had the efficacy, everyone would jump on that bandwagon. But sadly, going without food, whether it's for seventy-two or whatever number of hours, is just not a useful tool for curing cancer. Just like going without food for sixteen or whatever hours is not a useful tool for weight loss.

> **Hunger**
>
> Ending hunger is one of the first sustainable development goals that the world has agreed on, and in our country no one should have any misconceptions about what going without food for long hours can do. Other than the fact that it can prematurely kill you, it also increases school dropout rates, crime rates, disease rate, you name it, and only everything terrible is linked with it. And no amount of science or spirituality can put a positive spin to it.

Arif's confusion

Arif was a pulmonologist based in the US. He had three hard years at work during Covid. Now, with a bad stomach, poor fitness and weight gain, he had signed up for our program.

'I have read all your books,' he told me.

'How sweet,' I said.

'Now I am reading this,' he showed me another book on food. 'I read a lot.'

'Nice,' I said with my mouth and 'not so nice' in my mind.

'So, I wanted to ask,' he said, 'What's your take on IF? Because I have been on IF, low carb, high protein, it worked (roll your r's as you read that), but the weight bounces back, you know.'

Now, when you are talking to docs, you have to throw some jargon around, especially the first time around. So, I said, 'See, all these diets, they work till they don't. And in terms of studies, you have data that compares low carb to low fat, to IF, and none is better than the other. They just "work" because it helps reduce calories, that's the main mechanism. Also, now there's a study to show that people who routinely skip breakfast have a higher risk of certain gastro-intestinal cancers.[6] The trade-off is often not worth it.'

The poor guy had signed up for weight loss but was also facing indigestion, constipation, IBS-like symptoms and, to top it all, poor sleep. If I was at a talk, I would have said, '*If a diet has a name, it's bound to fail*,' but in a one on one, you have to explain a bit.

'Hmm,' he said.

'I will send you the link to the study,' I said. Something we have started doing of late. Some of our clients like to see, read stuff, or at least they pretend to.

> ### *Chhattees ka aakda*
>
> Mumbai has the best lingo on earth. One such way is to describe a relationship with a person as *'apun ka chhattees ka aakda hai'*. The person that you just cannot get along with is the person with whom you have *chhattees ka aakda* (number). In arranged marriages when *kundalis* are compared, if the 36 *gunas* match, then it's supposed to be a match made in heaven. Perfect on paper. But in lived experience, it's these couples that don't seem to get along at all, and so *chhattees ka aakda* is a euphemism for a strained relationship. Nothing wrong on paper, but *jamta nahi hai*. Because love isn't a calculation of risks and benefits, it is a meeting of hearts. When you marry people who have nothing in common but kundalis have a perfect score, you have set a disaster rolling. Remember this the next time you are reading some sciency stuff: just because it looks great on paper, it doesn't mean anything. A match made in heaven is put to test on earth. Similarly, a study under lab conditions will be actually tested in real life.

Why fasting doesn't work

Ok, here it is. All the reasons why fasting doesn't work:
1. The proof is in the physiology. And the physiology doesn't care whether it's a weekend or a weekday. All it cares for is that it allows you to live long, however sub-

optimally. So, when you go without food for long time periods – fourteen to sixteen hours – your body responds by lowering your energy output (baseline reset, which we will discuss in detail later). You get through your daily life and even your intense workouts with your body being on 'energy-save mode'. The only weight you lose is coming dominantly from your fat-free mass, muscles especially. So you are lighter on the scale and heavier on your feet. Feel me?

Also, bear in mind that physiology is not polite or kind to your weight-loss goals. Autophagy, a term often used to promote IF, is the body's mechanism to get efficient when resources are low. It doesn't love this. And ketones are a limited fuel, so they can let you do a light workout max. Anything intense and your body won't tolerate it, often leading to injuries. Maybe that's the reason why most fasting ads use just a walking model who keeps getting skinnier. This is also why OMAD (only one meal a day) plans will ask you to just do light walking max. Remember, youth and longevity are all about muscle strength and bone density, not skinny.

2. The proof is in the science. There is literally no conclusive evidence to show that fasting improves insulin sensitivity. Remember repeatability and reproducibility? In fact, eating only within a restricted feeding window means that people eat a lot more at one time or within that window than what they typically would, and that increases postprandial triglycerides. That's a big word for 'fat'. It can

therefore increase insulin resistance, the exact opposite of what you were hoping for. And when it comes to insulin sensitivity or heart health, exercise has actually proved to be an excellent intervention.

3. The proof is in the culture. I mean, exactly which fast was meant to take place all day, all night or all week with a two-day break? 5:2, or whatever? A fast where there is no restriction on alcohol and cigarettes, where there is no call to reflect on the impermanence of the body? This is not upavaas, it's bakwaas. The whole point of a traditional fast is that it is a time-bound practice where you celebrate community and diversity of food produce. Remove that and you just have a method of deprivation dressed up as a culture doll (more details under 'Fasting' in the chapter on cultural appropriation.)

4. The proof is in the lived experience. People who have been on a prolonged fasting, lose their sense of when to stop eating. This is the most common thing that my clients who were fasting would tell me – that they felt full and dull, no matter how little they would eat in the feeding window, and had no sense of satiety even if they ate a ton of food. It's a paradox that's hard to deal with in real time. For people who have always had a messed-up relationship with food, this becomes even more challenging. So, for all those who have been chubby, fat kids and teenagers, this just makes their body-image issues worse.

5. The proof is in the potty. The long hours of fasting, fourteen to sixteen, sometimes even twenty, often mean

more acidity, bloating and constipation. The excessive use of laxatives that fasting often requires can lead to a cycle of constipation and diarrhea (causing a loss of potassium that is linked to many complications, from poor digestion to excessive urination in the night, and in some rare cases, sudden heart failure also). Actually, there is no joy in lengthening your life span if you cannot have smooth, predictable bowel movements.

6. The proof is in the periods. The most common complaint with fasting among women, even for as little as a couple of months, is a messed-up cycle. One of the reasons is that in a limited eating window, you tend to not just eat larger meals but the diversity in your meals also takes a hit. And that can lead to poor micronutrient assimilation, especially that of iron, calcium, magnesium, and of vitamins like B12. This can lead to missed periods in young girls, scanty periods for those in their thirties and heavy flow for those around peri-menopause and menopause. It also makes hormonal headaches and migraines worse. Women, especially the young and fertile, as also those who are already pregnant or lactating, best stay away from IF.

Devil's advocate

But my trainer is looking amazing on IF. And why has my friend not complained of any symptoms?
The trainer is twenty-something, you are forty or older. If you look at your picture as a twenty-year-old, you were fairly skinny too. And athletic. Then you go down a path where there is an articleship in a CA's office or you study for some competitive exam, so you sit around a lot more than what you should for your average age. Then, at forty or sixty, you look different from those whose professions kept them on their toes in their twenties and thirties – the trainers, the actors, the dancers, etc. You can't grudge them that. And you cannot forget that the main role of food and even exercise is to make you better at what you do. And not to keep you in 'shape', but to keep you in good health. Happy and in harmony with the life you have built for yourself.

Also, just because your trainer or dietitian or whoever tells you something very confidently, don't believe it. Deep conviction in flawed beliefs is one of the signs of youth, just like good skin, smooth periods and bad boyfriends.

I went on a solo trek and my guide was a young twenty-year-old. He could rap, tell stories and make me laugh. Then he got comfortable enough to tell me his philosophy of life, 'Ma'am, if you do good, only good things happen to you. And if you do bad, bad things happen – if not today, then tomorrow.' For a moment I thought I should tell him that's not how life works. Bad things happen to perfectly good people all the time. And many wonderful things happen to terrible people too.

My grandfather used to say, every time he wanted us to know that his word is final, that he hadn't dyed his hair in the sun. To say that his greys was a sign of the life he had lived, and that his lived experiences gave him an edge over all that any one of us could possibly know through books, beliefs or theories.

I didn't say anything to my guide either. My hair too has earned its streaks of grey. I know that some things are best learnt by living, not by telling. Unfortunately, female clients (no matter how smart) tend to listen to everything that their male trainers tell them. We like being obedient, easy to work with, we seek approval, etc. It's a conditioning that all of us must question in good time.

But till then, we all must have one person in our lives with whom we have a non-transactional relationship (one you don't pay to be your trainer, dietitian or doctor), who's someone we know in real life (not someone we know from social media who answers our queries, likes our comments or retweets our replies), who's not our AI guide (who talks to us from a gadget) – someone in flesh and blood who has a *dil-se-dil ka rishta* with us.

It could be your mentor, neighbour, grandmother . . . anyone at all. And if this person feels that we are doing something extreme with our diets (even when we are loving the results and feeling on top of the world), then we should be ready to stop it. No questions asked. Stop the diet, not end the relationship.

In Marathi, the term for this is *'aapla manoos'*, which means *apna aadmi*, or 'main man', like they call it in the internet lingo, someone you can ask anything of, someone who will always be there for you, someone who makes you feel like you scored a 100 when you got out for a duck. Someone who can see your greatness before the world can see it and protects you from your own flaws and shortcomings. People who are invested in us can tell that something is going wrong even when we can't, and sometimes even when we think it's going great.

Broken window

In criminology, there's something called the 'broken window theory'. If a building has a broken window that has gone unrepaired for a long time, then it can become a breeding ground for serious crime over a period of time because it's a sign of neglect and that no one is in charge. People who have the connect with us that I have talked about can tell us that something is broken (small, but going unrepaired) even when no signs are present, either visibly or in blood reports. The broken-window approach is important. You get big things done by addressing the small stuff in a timely and effective manner. Small crimes, or small doubts about whether you are eating too much, or small needs such as wanting to fit into a smaller dress size, can lead to something more dangerous in the long run if not addressed right away.

> ## Baseline reset
> A mental and physiological adjustment to poorer day-to-day health that sets in over a period of time. Sub-optimal health becomes the new normal.

Dr Abhay, a famous haematologist, once told me about a case of a thirty-something woman he saw whose Hb was 3.4, and she had taken the train from Dahisar to his clinic in Bandra.

'How do they manage,' I asked?

'Oh, you will be surprised how the body adapts. I jumped out of my chair,' he said, 'but the woman said to me, "Doctor relax, *mi theek aahe*." If the drop is over a period of time, everything slows down and adapts to a lower level. Only if the drop is sudden, like an accident, do you crash. But if it's happening over many months or years, you are unfortunately fine.'

'Scary, but that's how resilient the human body is,' he concluded.

And if you are a woman, you need this *aapla manoos* even more. Because our baseline, when it comes to accepting poor outcomes with health, energy, sleep, etc., begins to shift at such a slow, steady speed that we can't keep pace. We continue living our lives, neglecting ourselves, and whipping ourselves into shape seems to be the only saving grace. But someone who knows us, cares for us, is able to spot the shift. It's just critical that we know them too, see them and hear them.

Here's another thing that I will tell you with the grey streaks in my hair and lines on my face. The fact is that every diet works. If 'works' is about getting you to fit into a smaller size of dress, lose weight and have some sense of achievement because of that. The question always is, at what cost?

3. Playing with single ingredients – sugar, dairy, gluten, etc.

'I don't touch sugar' is another flex, very common among the young these days. They are convinced that sugar is addictive and that it increases inflammation in our body and feeds cancer cells, or some such stuff. 'I am off sugar, salt, dairy and gluten' is the usual cocktail party refrain.

'Sugar makes the brain feel like it's on cocaine', she told me. She was a young, beautiful, rich brat engaged to one of my clients. She had refused kokum sherbet in my office because she was off sugar and was on her second cup of black coffee, impressed that our beans were single origin. 'Not bad haan, for aunty', she said to Pranay, whom I have worked with since he was a teenager and who is now in his mid-twenties.

He doesn't call me aunty, he calls me RD, but she called me aunty. *Arree itna pyar hai mujhse toh kokum pee*, but she was on a 'ccc' – caffeine, chocolate, constipation – diet. I was trying to make conversation, but it was getting difficult. She informed me that weed was therapeutic, Goyard was the new LV and that dark chocolate had more antioxidants than red wine. *'Aur koi mila nai kya,'* I wanted to ask my boy. My shrinking ovaries, bitter heart and old age were making it hard for me to hide my disappointment.

Swamiji of Parmarth Ashram in Rishikesh told me life is 'not fight or flight, it's fight or fine'. Some women cannot tolerate a word of nonsense after forty. Others, like me, develop an appetite for it. But I have had constant training really, my profession *mein kuchh karne* – or more importantly *karwane ke liye* – *bohot pyar se sab sun na padta hai.* That's my training ground, that's where you get the pulse of where and how far this will go, of the inclusions and exclusions to make in the diet plan. You learn that for long-term health you don't need to convert, you simply need to educate, advocate, regulate. That's when there is ownership, and therein lies success.

She continued, 'I was just telling Pranay that all I need from you is some advice to get sausage-like poop. And the PCO influencer I follow is recommending cocoa-sugar for good gut bacteria, because the bacteria in the brain is same as that in the gut. On most days I am like – take the protein, take the fat, take the fibre – because I honestly can't complicate life with food, etc. I am like eat to live, and not like Pranay's family who are forever discussing food. *Breakfast pe lunch ka discussion*. It's too much. I am like Virat Kohli, I don't care about taste.'

It was a *shola-tha-jal-bujha-hoon* kind of moment. 'So anything you tell me', she reassured me, 'I can do.' This wasn't a diet meeting, it was a meet-my-girlfriend meeting.

'I only have two problems – sausage-like poop and how to manage sugar cravings during PMS.'

'Ah! ok,' I said. 'Send me your three-day recall, I will look at it and make recommendations if I have any.'

The three-day recall is my saviour. I ask people to write that and most times I never have to hear from them again. In the rare instances that we do, we tell them what to do, and it always works. Telling people what to do must be rooted in their lives, their reality, or else you are just an #influencer and not a true-blue consultant (telling you what you already know for a fee :-)).

> **Box of sweets**
>
> Dr Joshi worked at Tata Memorial Hospital and, like all humans, wanted to lose weight. Seeing about forty to sixty patients a day was her regular routine, leaving her with little time and, more importantly, little bandwidth for anything else, be it planning meals or exercise. Weekends were dedicated to studying, writing, presenting and speaking at conferences, etc. One day, out of frustration, she decided that she was going to put up a notice in her OPD – 'Do NOT bring sweets for the doctor.' But her *mavshi* (assisting nurse) put her foot down. 'You can't do that,' she said. 'You don't have to eat all the sweets, just eat half a piece. We will send the rest to the children's ward, there are many other places where we can distribute sweets. It is the easiest and sweetest way for your patients to express gratitude after getting better. We can't take that joy away from them.' Great institutions are built on team work, where people are free to offer and take good advice without the hassle of hierarchy.

It's about context again

The thing is that when you cut out single ingredients based purely on their nutritional profile, it lands up being a massive misstep on your path to good health. Cutting out ghee for being a trans fat, cutting out sugar for being sugar, cutting out wheat for gluten, or cutting out rice for starch. The sensible thing to do is to always put them in context.

So, if we are to banish foods based on a single ingredient, we must check a few things: Is the study based on sugar in sherbet or on the consumption of sugar-sweetened beverages like colas or juices? How does this nutrient come into play in my specific cuisine? Has it always been part of my culture, like sugar in the dahi that my grandma gave as a blessing before big board exams or my first travel abroad? Is it in sync with the climate of where I live? Like a dahi–rice to cool me down or the sugar and salt in my nimbu sherbet to hydrate myself on a sports day?

Should I skip dairy?

- Not if it has been part of your cultural and regional food system.
- If you are intolerant or don't like milk and milk products, it's ok to not have them.
- But don't shift to 'alternatives' like almond or soy milk to make up for lost nutrients.

> - A diverse diet will more than take care of the absence of dairy in your diet.
> - Avoid industrial milk, support small farmers and cooperatives.

Essentially, when you cut stuff out of your day, and therefore life, you cut your connect with culture, cuisine and climate. Giving up sherbet because of a study on sugar-sweetened beverages is a big leap of faith. It's a big price to pay even if you are thin at the end of it. A simple way out of this confusion is to say the name of the said ingredient/nutrient/current villain in your native language. *Chini, sakhar, shaker, tumhare muh mein ghee shakkar.*

Nama smaran is a powerful tool even in spirituality, because it has the power to knock common sense back into your life. Hindu, Muslim, Sikh, Isai – everyone is into *japa mala* or beads or the rosary. Just take the familiar, friendly name of a food and know that you are safe. This is also why language is important when it comes to health, and when language is lost, cuisine and connect to community and culture are also lost. Enriched with hashtags, we then begin to lead impoverished lives.

Villainizing a single ingredient is like cutting a tree down to expand a road. You didn't just knock a tree down, you knocked down a home to butterflies, bees and birds. You knocked down shade to the migrant worker, the sight of a flower to a lover, the familiar sight to the ageing brain which could direct her home. And all you probably achieved was parking space for a car when you were actually hoping to make traffic move fast. Maybe you should just settle for cars moving at 30 kmph or less and make room for the public to walk, and root for better mass transport instead.

Ease of life

I had a client once tell me that he ran a few tests, saliva swabs and all the high-funda stuff and discovered that he was not allergic but intolerant to gluten. First of all, I don't have even *one* rupee *ka* faith in these tests, but that rant is for another book. He was of course wanting to lose weight so he went off rotis and ate only kuttu rotis. '2 p.m. to 8 p.m., my diet is clean.' Yeah, clean eating is a thing. Just like not eating before 2 p.m. is. 'Then post 11 p.m., I just get too many cravings. But I try to eat clean only, so I eat a packet of digestive biscuits, and for salt some makhana and kabhi if I feel like having a sweet, I squeeze all the syrup out and eat a rasgulla.'

'*Digestive ka gluten* you are not intolerant to?' I asked.

'Shit!' he said. '*Kya pakda!*' He got up and shook my hand. I wanted to weep, though.

Fully functional people doing random things – oh, the grip the food and weight-loss industry has, even over the geniuses, is quite something. This guy had built a factory from scratch, and at fifty-eight he now had over 6,000 employees. Building an empire from nothing is an act of determination, drive and discipline, but it comes at the cost of neglecting one's health. It shouldn't, but it does. You wait in people's offices endlessly, you do your own paperwork tirelessly, you walk 17-20 km in a day when you run out of bus fare. The trials and tribulations are endless.

The whole ease of business only starts after a certain set point, but till that time it's all uphill. At least it has been for this generation. Their children can now aspire to leave the office at 5 p.m., play tennis and have a life – not that this includes eating right, but again that's for another book ;-). First-generation entrepreneurs always have it rough; their wealth costs them their waistline. And it's not because they are greedy people who don't know when to stop eating or lack the will or desire for good health; it's the twenty-odd years of negligence or other priorities that take a toll. Their success nevertheless must be celebrated. **Hustling is hard on the health**, and the only sustainable approach now is to nurture the body back into good shape.

Devil's advocate

But then why do some people feel better after going #dairyfree or #glutenfree?

'Everyone is gluten and dairy free these days, kya?' asked one of my clients. Rochelle was a free-spirited young girl, making her career in Canada. She was an East Indian from Vasai and she loved the fact that my roots are in Vasai too and that our ancestral home is at Parnaka. 'Then you know my fav food,' she said. 'Bhujing chicken,' I replied. 'Yes!' she exclaimed. 'And the second one is?' 'Chaha,' I guessed right again. This mtg was already going well.

'If I get my fully loaded chaha (sugar and milk and tea leaves boiled to death), then the rest of the day, I am happy to not eat anything at all. But on shifting to Canada, I have noticed that I have gotten dairy intolerant. Full day I am burping, in dresses my stomach is showing, the other day my mom asked me on video call, what happened to your skin? Full break outs I have. Must be dairy only I figured. But then chai without milk I cannot imagine and with soy, almond milk toh it stinks, so now what to do?' She asked.

Dr Gursimran, one of my clients, is a gastroenterologist based in Pittsburgh, and an alumnus of Cleveland Clinic. During an Insta LIVE with me on IBS, he spoke about how kids who get a bad stomach during exams get a bad rep. *'Haan, kuch nahi, bas natak hai,'* because after exams their stomachs are just fine and they are playing and all. 'But what we don't realize is that they are not pretending, the stress can affect digestion, cause pain, gas, bloating, nausea. And once that stress is over, your digestion returns to normal. We must also ask why every kid across the globe says, stomach is hurting and not head or hand? Because that's what actually hurts.'

Was Rochelle stressed? Yes. Not every girl has relationship stress. But the stress of making it on foreign soil in an era of economic instability and war, is real. As is not having the luxury of a fully functioning kitchen. Long meal gaps, eating the same batch of food for ten days, eating out of boredom, not to forget, eating nothing and starting the day with chai. Sometimes, all you need is a life that is free of repetitive errors. So, we added a date on waking up, fixed the long gaps with a fruit or nuts that she would carry in her bag, got her to cook fresh twice in a week, and planned for meals out so that they were not last-minute boredom decisions. And voila, the stomach no longer bloated with the cup of chai. Sometimes, it's the little things you do – the timing, the negligence, the phase of life and not necessarily the dairy. Or gluten for that matter.

But then why do some people actually feel better after going #dairyfree or #glutenfree? Because the "nocebo effect" is real. You may experience negative effects of an inert substance just because you are expecting to feel worse. So, the thing to do, as usual, is to do the first things first. Check on the basics – eating on time? Exercising too much or nothing? Sleeping too late? And work on fixing those first. Because going #glutenfree #dairyfree will not resolve the problems that these bring. And over time, you may have to bring in many more #free to your life. Eventually, your diet gets so restricted that instead of tackling stresses of youth better, you feel overwhelmed by them.

But if you do address the underlying issues first, there is a good chance that your tolerance will improve, if not immediately, then over time. Having said that, in rare cases the intolerance to these substances is real, in which case simply avoid them. You don't have to replace these single ingredients with alternatives though.

2

Pseudo-cultural trends

Cultural appropriation

My client whatsapped me a news clip that read 'Mantralaya to serve kokum juice to all visitors', and captioned it '*tera jalwa*'. This is my advertising client who believes that by not being smart about endorsements (i.e., by choosing to not do them at all) I have lost a ton of money. He believes that I should have a slice of pie from the 10,000-crore ghee market, from the makhana madness, from all these startup kids putting kokum now in every soap or cream, and from five-stars who are now serving local dishes for breakfast and not just cold cuts, etc.

On his part, he has given up his corner office, quit his ad job ('*jhooth bol bol ke thak gaya*') and now teaches full time and mentors kids in a premier arts college. He has also scored a side gig to teach classes on creativity in short-term courses at IIM-A. He has signed off his sea-facing Worli flat to his ex, has paid in advance for his children's education abroad and now divides his time between teaching, looking after his dog and giving free advice to people like me who don't take it.

Wealth is like health. You get to define what it means for you. Does it set you free to pursue your calling? Does it matter what others think about your choice? Is it taking away more than what it brings you? You alone are in a position to answer these questions, and the answers may very well change with time. A sprawling sea-facing apartment may lose its sheen compared to the sight and sounds of ideas of the new generation of students.

Your flex now could be that you give shape and form to ideas. Because every good idea is only a pitch and execution away from greatness. 'People don't invest in products, they invest in stories.' That's what your Dalal Street guy is going to tell you if you want to raise money. Tell a story, tell a good one. Tell one that is scalable, tell one of legacy.

Kokum sherbet is that story. The product is kokum, the pitch is that it's a digestive aid and hydrating. But the *baap* is the execution – the sherbet. The best way to create value with the product is to get the execution right – *kya bolte usko*, build an easy-to-use interface.

Kaun kiya yeh execution possible, yeh interface itna smooth? The collective wisdom of our land, of our women – this is our indigenous wealth. The kokum fruit is not just used in sherbets but also as flavouring in dals and sabzis. Even its application as a drink is not just in sherbet, where it's mixed with water, but also in saar, where it's mixed with buttermilk to stoke the appetite. It is also used in the form of butter to heal cracks on the heels.

So, the fruit of the Western Ghats is like a good movie. A good movie is made on two tables – the writing table and the editing table. Every person from the industry knows this. So, to create value you must first flesh out your idea, and then you must mercilessly cut out the parts that are not relevant to the story you are telling. So, the seed is not there in the drink, the fruit is not a part of the butter, but the seed is, and so on.

But to the diet industry, everything is worth its weight only in profits, not in the value it creates. And so the latest on the bandwagon is what my ad guy calls 'cultural appropriation', and I call 'pseudo-cultural'. It is about picking up indigenous ideas or ingredients and pitching them for weight loss/cleansing /killing cancer, etc., and the execution consists of just consuming a lot of it at one time. If-it's-good-a-lot-of-it-must-be-great kind of a funda. So the interface isn't smooth, it isn't even scalable, but it is milkable until the next trend.

That's also where the trends of 'clean' eating or even 'satvik' eating come in. Monotony rules, diversity is shown the door. If you take a spice like haldi, or a seed like methi, and enter any Indian kitchen, you find hajaar ways of using these ingredients. But where is the value in the small roles they play in ten different foods? Capitalism means *ek hero ingredient ke naam pe dus cheez bechna*. So you now have a haldi pill, a haldi chai, a haldi chocolate (vomit). Spend money, buy #immunity, #guthealth #weightloss #mentalhealth.

The weight-loss industry uses ingredients out of context, focuses only on a single characteristic of each ingredient and makes it what it is not. Black or white with no room for nuance, much like being on X. It's like watching a movie where the writing is bad, the main character has no arc, and everyone else's role is diminished.

One of my clients, a successful founder, was on one of those diets. Soaked seeds in the morning, followed by jeera water, haldi water and moringa powder. Lunch was *quinoa ka khichdi*, dinner *millet ka roti*. And *baja hua hein neend and pet ka band*. He wondered why, because he ate so 'clean'.

'That's the problem, *gandagi chahiye thoda*'. He was from IIT-B, but my joke didn't land.

The thing is that while appropriating culture and traditions and packaging them with hashtags is a new trend, it works because of the old problem of intelligent people putting their common sense aside when it comes to food. Or weight loss or health. New practice, old problem. That people are willing to do anything, anything to lose weight. So low cal, low carb, high protein, good fat *kar liya*, *sab* permutations and combinations done and dusted, now culture and ancient traditions *se khelo*.

Sapta dhatu

The Indian belief is that the food we eat nourishes the *sapta dhatu*, or the seven layers of our body – *rasa, rakta, mamsa, medha, asthi, majja* and *shukra*. Loosely translated, rasa is digestive juices, ratkta is blood, mamsa is muscles, medha is fat, asthi is bones, majja is bone marrow and shukra is sexual fluids. When we fail to eat properly or fall prey to quick fixes, these dhatus don't get the nourishment they need to stay healthy. If you have lost weight earlier but couldn't keep it off, you can think of it as the revenge of the sapta dhatus.

This is the typical weight loss where you say *face se glow chala gaya*, but arms and belly are still fat, or the one where you weigh lesser on the scales but your aunty is asking you why you look sick. The right proportions of food, i.e., not overdoing any one ingredient, are responsible for all the seven dhatus receiving their due. That way, you lose weight in a sustainable manner, lose fat, build better bone density and musculature, regulate your periods and address your micronutrient deficiencies without an injection of vitamin D or B12. It is the type of weight loss where people ask you how much have you lost, 10 kg or 15 kg? And you confess that it's not even a kilogram on the scale, and they decide that you are just lying.

1. Gut cleanses/detox

The *davaa* that is created for the *dard* that unsustainable diets bring. Now you have diets for diets that don't work. I told you that the world of dieting is getting nastier because people are now on many diets at one time. They are fasting and eating only protein, and that too only through 'Ayurvedic' or plant-based foods like zoodles with asparagus and mushrooms in a Buddha bowl.

Or only keto, fat and low carb, dollops of avocado and kale on the side or whatever version of that. The more unrealistic, the better. Caffeine unlimited, and the cream that they put on Starbucks coffee is only 47 kcals please, so it has to be ok. When you go through days and weeks of this, you break. So does your gut integrity, your resolve and your common sense. Then you treat yourself over the weekend to chocolate cake, chhole bhature and chips. Some wine and shots on the side because *apne #bhaikabudday* or some other equally worthy occasion like #groomdoom or *#dulhankigang*, or you are simply chilling with friends.

Come Monday morning and you are on a #gutcleanse. The dream of the #gutreset allows you the nightmare of the weekend where you eat and drink all that you don't need because you are going to clean up anyway. In an alternative world, Krishna is telling Arjun that not just the words you speak or the arrows you shoot, but what you binge-eat over the weekend cannot be recalled, much less cleansed.

But in this world, *gut cleanse is the new way to detox the age-old guilt.* Where even the food that you used to enjoy once, you cannot anymore. If only you were on a more realistic diet, just a meal of chhole bhature or a samosa or a cake with your friends would have been more than enough. But now that you are fully *chootoing* after being trapped in multiple diets ka combo for the week, one thing doesn't satiate, and bingeing *toh banta hai.* Once again, you should go for the middle path, or the *suvarna madhyam.* Liberate your diet a bit and restrict your cheating a bit instead of swinging to the other extreme of detox/cleanse.

Truth be told, that cleanse of yours is just as toxic as your weekend binge. And you stand to lose confidence, composure and common sense in the long run. Not worth it, not at all. But sometimes I see people doing a cleanse just because their friend is doing it too.

My 70-year old neighbour greeted me in the lift one day. 'Oh, good I met you, I did a cleanse and I was just thinking about you. That you will be so angry.' (A lot of my friends, clients and neighbours only think of me as 'oh she will be so angry').

'Why did you do it?' I asked.

My neighbour is a very sensible girl, a producer who knows where to put her money.

'Oh, all my friends were doing it.'

So it's not a twenties problem, this is a sangat problem. 'You have mad friends,' I told her.

'I know,' she said.

During Covid, people would do wine parties on screen, and it has now turned to drinking salt water, cayenne pepper or laxative tea, while puking offline and supporting each other online. Of course, you can pay millions and also go to spas and detox farms to do the same. 'Better than paying lakhs to you and eating dal–chawal,' said one of my clients. Touché.

Reduce the variance

Variance is a mathematical concept that measures, of course, variability. In simpler terms, it measures how far you are spread out from the *suvarna madhyam*. The thing with high variance is that it is the hallmark of inefficiency – whether in sports, economics, work or diet. You spend the entire week being off carbs, salt, calories, etc. Come weekend you can't stop eating those; you don't even keep out the ultra-processed food products. From two-minute noodles to chocolate cookies, from pav bhaji to ice-cream, from sharab to shawarma, everything is on the menu.

The variance is too high. Some people don't even wait for a week to transition from one extreme to another, they do it daily, being very strict during the day and bingeing in the night. Intraday trading is dangerous, whether with diet or money. So, have a fair and square policy with low variance, where all food groups are represented and all occasions, special and routine, have a place.

The thing is, a detox for those in their forties and above can even put their kidneys, heart and other critical organs at risk because of the loss of electrolytes, due to the diarrhoea, vomiting and the dehydration it causes. The whole point, after all, is to age well and look good. So it just can't be left for the Insta reels to say things like 'These are not my wrinkles but my medals'. You must also learn to be mature with age.

In real life, if it's a 42- or 52-inch waistline and not a 32- or a 28-inch one, it's ok. You can reduce it to under 36 inches in a year or two, steadily and sustainably. Without the drama and delusion that detox brings, shrinking to half in a week and expanded to double in three days flat. 'Even normal speed will get you there' is one of my favourite Border Roads Organisation (BRO) road signs, and that applies to our bodies too.

Gut doesn't need cleansing

Ek hi dil hai kitni baar jeetoge, ek hi gut hai kitni baar cleanse karoge? Instead, learn the term 'health-washed'. Like brainwashed, where logic is put aside to accept a narrative as fact, health-washing is where an extreme practice is pushed as a healthy one. Like cleansing, where you first wash your sins with mixtures of salts, oils, warm water and other such 'detoxifying' agents. The nausea, loosies and giddiness it creates is celebrated as 'cleansing' and not seen as threatening. But they are, to good health. Health, you must remember, is in the balance.

And this may break your heart, but just like how you don't need to send ugly teddy bears on V Day, you don't need to drink up pink, yellow, green potions to cleanse your system. Actually, you don't need any external aid to clean your system, barring bathing, brushing and rinsing your mouth after food. Everything else is just full time-pass. And costly. Not just to the inheritance of money but to the wealth of flora and fauna that resides right from your mouth to your anus.

We inherit good microbes from our parents, take a lifetime to build on it and then risk washing it away with all the 'cleansing'. Irrespective of whether they are called '*kriyas*', 'detoxes' or 'gut resets', they will take away the good with the bad. The body has natural ways to deal with the bad – it is called gut permeability; an inbuilt system to keep the good protected from the bad microbes. It also has the liver, the kidneys, lungs and skin, which constantly detoxify the body without making any fuss, and for free. Free, free.

Good health and a good gut are built by the routine practices of eating home food, exercising and sleeping on time. And the gut is really just a stylish way to address your digestive system. In the nineties, girlfriends were called '*jaan*' or '*jaanu*', now they are called 'baby', but *Urdu ho ya angrezi, hai toh future biwi hi.*

The thing to remember is that every cleanse puts you on the path to the next one in a couple of months. This is because a depleted gut flora causes bloating and gas, and then we fix it by eating a very limited diet. Most things begin to leave our plate; the stuff we grew up eating now troubles us. This is because the bacteria needed to digest and break down food has been flushed down the drain.

Instead of these cycles, build a diverse diet – one that your grandma will smile upon. Because diversity breeds diversity.

#guthealth

The more protein from 'products', the lesser the fibre from natural sources (remember what I told you about the food matrix). And so, in the recent past, you must have seen the rise and rise of the hashtag #guthealth. So, you ate all the protein diligently, and now you are taking more time in the bathroom and are considering a gut cleanse. But before that, how about some fibre as a prebiotic? Maybe this one drink or pill can fix your constipation and flatulence?

Who would have imagined that the likes of Isabgol would run ads with celebrity endorsement, with airport and highway placements? *'Kabz aap ko hota hai par pata sab ko hota hai.'* When Rishi Kapoor delivered this line, it reminded me all over again why all budding actors are taught to watch him emote in songs.

But coming back to the point, one product creating a market for another product is the best kind of business ever. And you will find many influencers telling you that all you need is protein, fibre and omega (not the watch, the fat). I say, learn from them. That conviction is all you need to propose to your next girlfriend, pitch your next idea, plan your next home décor.

2. Fasting

One of the prime examples of cultural appropriation is the new trend of fasting. We already discussed IF in the previous chapter, but it's also portrayed as being 'part of our culture/an age-old practice/*pehle hum din mein do meals hi khate the*', etc. So I want to touch upon fasting in this section, but from the cultural point of view.

One of the pillars of Hinduism is the idea that while everything is turbulent and unpredictable, there is one thing that is constant, one's *shraddha* or devotion to the higher reality; and hopefully, with that, the realization of all that is impermanent. *Bhasmantam shareeram* – eventually the body is reduced to ashes. Coming from the land of yoga, intellectually at least, we all buy into that. But emotionally, our attachment to the body is strong.

Six stages of the body

Vedanta philosophy categorizes the body into six distinct stages through the life cycle of a person. Please bear in mind that the English translations are loose, to say the least, but you will very much get the drift.

Asti – Existence. The body exists, right from the time you are in the womb.

Jayate – It is born. And now can have a life of its own.

> *Vardhate* – It grows. The body grows with time. The naturally anabolic stage.
>
> *Viparinamite* – It changes or matures. Whether it's with puberty or age.
>
> *Apakshiyate* – It deteriorates. Yes, that does happen with time. The naturally catabolic stage of the body.
>
> *Vinaschiyati* – It dies. Hopefully with ripe old age and nothing else, but die it surely will.
>
> This is also what YOLO means. That you will get to experience all of this exactly once in your life. So don't be in the past or in the future in your head, stay in the present and make the most of it.

Whenever it's Ramzan, Navratri or Paryushan, my inbox is flooded with 'What can I do to lose weight during this time' messages. *Iss hamam mein, hum sab nange hai.* Fasting, in fact, is about rethinking everything that consumes us, be it the obsession with weight loss, the body or the food we eat. It has four pillars:

1. *Swadhyaya* – Study of the self. It was meant as a practice that honed the mind, body and senses. It meant for us to go inside, to connect with the formless, nameless, genderless, all-pervasive life-force. And, sorry to break your heart, but no fast was meant for #detox, #cleanse, #weightloss. Which is why, in Sanskrit, it's called 'upa-

vaas' – being in proximity to the supreme being – and not called by a term that translates into 'guaranteed weight loss'.

2. *Tapa* – Voluntary renunciation (of certain foods, for example). It was meant as a practice of introducing diversity to one's diet. To appreciate all that nature offers as food and to understand that health and harmony come from diversity. So, if Lent encouraged followers to go #meatfree and include more veggies in the diet, then Paryushan brought the millets and pulses into the spotlight by removing green veggies from the plate. Navratri or Ekadashi placed emphasis on tubers like suran and arbi, millets like rajgeera, etc., with generous offering of nuts. And Ramzan on dates, fresh fruits and homemade milkshakes. Diversity is the key here, not deprivation.

3. *Maitri* – Friendship and celebration of seasons, rituals and family bonds. Essentially, fasting was a practice that allowed you to understand that variety is the spice of life. The fast didn't come randomly but followed a calendar that was based in a deeper understanding of nature. The celebratory meals were, and are, for everyone, the ones who fast and the ones who don't. The ones who believe and the ones who don't. No one gets a lecture on fasting at the celebrations, everyone is goaded to eat more.

4. *Karuna* – Compassion. Any grandmother who follows roza will tell you that it is a reminder that no one should go hungry, and hence the practice of *anna daan*, almost on a daily basis, during Ramzan. In fact, irrespective of

the name or the origin of the fast, if one developed a headache, nausea or weakness, it wasn't an endorsement of the effectiveness of the practice (wow, toxins are coming out) or something that one must endure, but an indication that the fast must be stopped and normal routine should be resumed.

Which is also why the very old, the very young, the pregnant, the ailing, women on periods, lactating mothers, etc., were discouraged from fasting. The idea was to be sensitive to pain and to understand it, not endure it. And to lead a life where one doesn't cause pain to oneself or to others around.

P.S. – *Hatha Yoga Pradipika*, one of the guiding texts of yoga, says that anyone on the path of yoga should stay away from all extremes, including fasting.

But isn't fasting a spiritual practice?

'What do you think, Rujuta?' asked one of my clients. She had just been to an ashram, taken *diksha* from her guru and done a course which she said had re-engineered, re-imagined and re-birthed her. I was happy for her, but she was conflicted. The guru wanted her to eat only twice a day, and after her battle with weight and self-image for over twenty-five years, she had just begun to eat correctly. She started her day with raisins, ate breakfast, ate a fruit in between, had lunch, a snack, and then went on to have dinner. And she had never felt lighter or looked better. The migraines had gone, the waist was narrow; sleep, even poop, was better, but now this *dharma sankat*. 'You think I should let go of this body trap and follow spirituality? Eat only twice and focus on my breathing instead of food if I get hungry?'

You know, the only reality check the world needs is kindness and compassion. It's even good for business. And I learnt this a long time ago. So, if one of my clients comes back with something unrealistic for their daily lives that is recommended by their favourite friend, guru or trainer, I don't put the advice or the advisor in a bad light. Ridiculing doesn't work, reasoning does. After all, we are just trying for that sweet middle, the *suvarna madhyam*.

In Sarika's case, I reminded her that the guru was beyond the realm of the body but that she was planning for IVF; we needed to nurture her body. 'Sarika, it won't work. What a mahatma can achieve, we can't. And that is why even in the ashram, there is a café, isn't there? He may instruct you to eat only twice, but the café on the premises is open all hours so that followers can be gentle on themselves. Continue what is working for you, eat the way you have been eating, and integrate the spiritual practices you have learnt in the ashram. But don't give up your food, dreams and ambitions for it.'

And as a footnote, I would like to add – though I didn't say this to Sarika – that in the Sant and Warkari *parampara* of Maharashtra, it's *'pehila potoba, nantar vithoba'*. It means that all spirituality talk is humbug when the stomach is empty.

I told you; I will repeat it: Whether it's health, science or spirituality, the ones who watch it up close and personal have a view that is rooted in practicality, far away from the narrative of miracles that claim to cure all that ails the mind and body.

3. Seeds and spices

Akele nahin, ek saath

There was a time when people would dutifully avoid spices, '*Hum bas saada khaana khate hai*, no masala for us.' Today they start the day with shots of haldi, jeera, methi daana and what not. Traditional foods, yes, but consumed in novel ways set by the food and weight-loss industries. On my recent UK trip, I stayed at a posh hotel but took the room-only rate. The server, however, would send me the shot of the day for free. One day it was a turmeric shot and the next day a cinnamon one. *Ek zamane mein* it would be soup of the day, and you would need to pay for it. Or if you were a pretty girl, a guy would buy you a drink, a shot of vodka maybe. Now routine girls like me get sent spice shots for free.

Truth be told, our collective wisdom of using seeds or spices is thousands of years old. Their use, in predetermined combinations and proportions, has been orally transmitted for generations. They were used to enhance the flavour of food and to improve assimilation of nutrients in combination with other ingredients, and never consumed in large quantities by themselves. Essentially, this took care of the naturally existing anti-nutrients in food (which come in the way of nutrient absorption) and ensured that food was used and not abused as therapy.

For example, haldi was always used with fat, like in a tadka in oil or with milk, and not as haldi shots in water. Similarly, the use of methi dana or curry patta in tadka, making flaxseed chutney, and so on, was part of regular kitchen practices so that you consume them in the right proportion. We undervalue the priceless wisdom of our women folk and their selfless labour in our kitchens and land up paying a big price (monetarily and health wise) by following diet trends. If a little is good, then a lot is not better. And your dadi did know better than your dietician.

> **Aliv seeds**
>
> After I wrote about aliv seeds in *Indian Superfoods*, it was like the world had discovered them. Soon after, I would find people taking garden cress seeds soaked in water on an empty stomach in an attempt to improve their hair growth and Hb levels.
>
> The seeds are a source of folic acid, iron, etc., yes, but their magic is in the process – the soaking in the nariyal pani, the mixing in ghee, jaggery and coconut, cooking it all on low heat in an iron *kadhai* and rolling them into a laddoo upon cooling. But the fear of weight gain would keep them away from ghee, jaggery and coconut. And then just the seeds would mean stomach distress and little or no impact on Hb levels.

The best way for the assimilation of nutrients without any undue load on the GI tract is to keep up with the time-tested combinations. And this is not just about aliv seeds, it is true even for cinnamon shots, methi shots, whatever shots. The blood sugar-lowering properties are in the full combination not in a singular ingredient. And what matters is the complete meal and not individual nutrients.

Think of each spice like a person. A real person comes with the good and the bad. There are environments like families, teams, friends, etc., that enable the good. And then, if by chance you meet this person without his wife or outside his work environment, you don't really like him any more. The proportion and the setting in which he was good is taken away, and now that you have a lot of him, and it begins to make you feel restless, uncomfortable, stressed. Experienced this?

Well, spices are exactly like that. Too much of them (shots and pills), then say hello to acne, missed periods and bloating. Too little of them, and say bye bye to smooth skin, pain-free periods and a flat stomach.

The spice box

What can a humble spice dabba found in every single Indian kitchen teach us about health and nutrition? That there are a variety of spices we use daily, that we use them in small quantities and that we mostly use them in cooking. However, if we go by the latest fads of using spices, which mostly consists of adding them to water and drinking it first thing in the morning, we will be refilling this dabba every few days and not every few weeks, as we usually do.

Antinutrients

One client recently told me that he was eating soaked methi seeds daily to lower his HbA1c. He was upset that it hadn't worked even when he was advised that eating them on an empty stomach would mimic insulin. The thing is that all natural foods, in addition to having therapeutic properties, also have something called anti-nutrients – naturally existing molecules like oxalates, phytates, tannins, lectins, goitrogens, etc. – which can come in the way of nutrient assimilation.

This means that they can actually prevent the active or therapeutic ingredient that you seek from the food from reaching you, even if you ate a lot of it. Now, you can't remove the anti-nutrient, but you can neutralize its effect by soaking, sprouting, cooking and combining them with other foods like they were always meant to be.

Consuming any spice or seed like a pill is therefore not effective. But as a part of your dietary pattern of eating them in a tadka, as a chutney, laddoo, etc., remains a sane and safe way to regulate blood sugars, control BP, beat obesity and whatnot (because regular home-cooked food just works, and works like magic). Whereas raw, by itself and on an empty stomach is the ghettoization of nutrients, and whether it's people or nutrients, ghettos are just a poor way to live or eat.

4. Millets

The new maida

Sometimes we begin a reintroduction of all things ancient in our diet without context. Millets have gone through something like that. I could write a whole book on their goodness, but there's a good chance that you may already know it all – they are rich in micronutrients, they are dense in fibre, they can help regulate blood sugars, blood pressure and even help with weight loss. And with that information, millets are the new – and it breaks my heart to say this – maida.

Everything that was once made with maida – biscuits, cakes, breads, noodles, etc. – is now being made with millets so that more profit can be made by positioning it as healthy. But as we now know, good health isn't about replacing x with y; it is about understanding the context, and then, if needed, reintroducing it in our daily diets.

The makeover of millet

I was at a NITI Aayog event where there was a panel discussion on millets. The chief of NITI Aayog spoke about how calling millets 'coarse cereals' was a misstep and gave them the tag of being a poor man's food. He said they were now called 'nutri-cereals', which reflected the reality of millets better. He went on to wonder though, if policymakers

> were doing enough to ensure that millet awareness didn't just mean shifting millets from the poor man's plate to the rich man's. Millet awareness, he said, must translate into more land under cultivation (important for climate mitigation), and entry of millets in the PDS (for beating malnutrition), and shouldn't get reduced to #millets. Because real change starts from the soil and the ones who toil on it. Farm-food-fitness are interlinked in more ways than you can think.

As a Maharashtrian, I have grown up eating bhakri, or millet roti, at one meal daily. In the farming communities, it is bhakri for lunch. In working Marathi households, it's typically bhakri for dinner, as they taste nicer when consumed hot. Also, because we now lack the skill or competence that is required to make them in a way where they taste great even when they are no longer hot.

To move the bhakri to dinner time is a practical, sensible adaptation. One rooted in ground reality. Adaptations of all good things have to be thought through, or else they are #epicfail. Anyone who works in policymaking understands the glocal concept. Just because it's a great policy that worked wonders somewhere doesn't mean you can pick it up and dump it here, too. You will have to make revisions or adopt only a part of it so that the outcomes are as desired.

If the outcome you wish out of millets is a lean body, great figure, better Hb levels, lower blood sugar, blood pressure, etc., then replacing all things maida with millets won't help. Nor will it help that you now have your gaucamole with millet chips, your stew with millet noodles or your veggies with millet pasta or the lettuce with pearl millet.

It means that you must learn how to roll a bhakri and have it with your sabzi. Or you pick an easier recipe and make a ragi dosa instead. Or you could make the easy lassi, kheers or laddoos with millets. The problem is that we want the millets without the baggage they come with – the labour, the sugar, the ghee, the pulses – only because these other ingredients are not the flavour of the month. But that's not how digestion works. This baggage that it comes with are actually agents that make it easier for your body to assimilate the goodness of millets. Without this, it is just another trend that is waiting to get replaced by yet another.

A lesson from Vishal Bharadwaj

Vishal and Rekha Bharadwaj had come over for dinner, and I was telling Rekha ji how I can still hear the ghazal that she sang at one of her live programs at Prithvi theatre. Small, intimate audience, with hardly any instruments and no mic. *Gulon mein rang bhare* was the ghazal, and it sounded even better than Mehdi Hassan's, even though she sang it exactly like he did. Some things are so precious that they should not be changed, and yet, like a time-tested recipe, when you make it, your individuality shines through. VB then asked me if I had heard his version, and I said no, sorry, I hadn't. He then went on to narrate how this was one of his favourite ghazals and he had set the tune for the *antara* in his own style. Arijit Singh was supposed to record it. He had heard it, loved it and had said, 'Let me go out for some fresh air and I will come back and record it.' Ten, twenty, thirty minutes later, there was no sign of Arijit, and when VB had called him, he had said, 'I have left the studio, I can't sing this version because my guru always sang the OG.'

VB said he had to get his team to slowly warm up Arijit to listen to his tune, allow it to grow on him and to understand the thought process behind it. Only then was it recorded. It took months, but the VB version sung by Arijit is beautiful too. The next time you want to take a millet and turn it into something creative or take a wild vegetable and turn it into a mocktail, ask yourself – are you a genius like VB, because even he left the *mukhada* of the ghazal unchanged. The magic is in the familiarity, not in the creativity.

Eating millets the right way

1. *Eat millets according to season*
   Eating seasonal not only ensures easy availability of nutrients at just the time they are needed, but it also ties in beautifully with farming practices and crop cycles. Here is a quick guide to which millets work best for which season:

- Bajra is for the winters – eat it with jaggery and ghee
- Jowar is better for summers – eat it with a chutney
- Ragi/nachni is eaten all year round, but especially during the rains, and can even be turned into dosa, laddoo, porridge, etc.
- The lesser-known millets are usually linked to change of season and are mostly tied to festivals – millets like raajgira, samo, kuttu and others.

This is also the reason you shouldn't use ready-made multi-grain flour, as it goes against the time-tested wisdom of eating as per the season.

2. *Eat millets in the right food combinations*
   Combining millets with pulses, spices and fats ensures that limiting amino acids are compensated for, protein quality and digestibility improved and the effect of antinutrients reduced. Millets that are particularly hard to digest, like bajra, even come with rules – e.g., always have them with a dollop of makhan or an extra teaspoon of ghee and never without jaggery. One can't but marvel at dadis and nanis *ke gharelu nuskhe* and their saral, sasta and sundar methods of turning every meal into a joy, long after it's been consumed.

Listen to your wife

I was once on a solo holiday in Haridwar, staying at a boutique homestay. It was the last week of December, but before the New Year madness. It was beautiful and quiet. On the table next to me for dinner was a couple, ten to fifteen years older than me. I was enjoying their conversation, it was full of warmth, of temples they had visited, the street food they tried, the perfect weather, etc. Then the wife told the husband to eat jaggery with the ragi roti they were having. 'You didn't eat it in the morning also,' she said.

'I just want to know the logic,' he replied.

'You don't need to know everything, Rajat, just eat it,' she said. I was loving this. Then I overheard that they were leaving for Delhi within the next twenty minutes for a meeting in the morning.

'Oh no,' I thought to myself, and I said aloud to them that this was the most romantic dinner I had ever witnessed.

'Oh! I won't hear the end of it now,' the husband said to me, while the wife winked at me playfully.

Sometimes I talk too much, and I said to the husband, 'You must just listen to your wife, you know, about the jaggery.'

'I am an engineer; I need to understand why jaggery with ragi roti.'

'It's a hygiene practice, like how you would calibrate instruments before use daily, clean vessels before producing the next batch, check brakes before you go on a long drive.'

> I had no idea what kind of engineer he was, *toh jitna example aata tha, sab bol diya*. 'The thing is, when you eat jaggery with ragi, or any millet for that matter, you reduce errors, you ease out digestion.'
>
> 'See, this I understand. Shikha, you could have told me this,' he said to his wife.
>
> 'She doesn't need to, you must just always listen to your wife,' I winked back at her. Honestly, I always pray that husbands don't listen to their wives and kids to their mothers, because that's the only way people like me can stay in business.

3. *Eat millets in all forms*

   The diversity in the ways we can consume millets is staggering. They can be germinated and fermented for satva, kheer or porridge; they can be soaked and cooked to make khichdis; they can be made into bhakris and roasted to make laddoos. All this ensured that there was no taste fatigue or boredom in eating nutritious, healthy food.

4. *Don't replace all grains with millets*

   Lastly, know that millets are not a replacement for rice and wheat. At least not a complete replacement. Again, it comes back to sustainability and common sense. So, continue with the rice and/or wheat for normal consumption, but don't forget the weekly bhakri and the seasonal laddoos and porridge.

Making a millet bhakri

Is there a way for us to eat millets where we can access all of their nutrients and create no ecological waste? Yes, there is. And it is a well-known one. Just use your millets and convert them into a bhakri/rotla. Eat them with a sabzi, dal or chutney.

I know that it's tough to make rotlas and that they break, so I am going to share a kitchen secret on how to roll them without breaking. Use warm water when kneading the atta, and then hand-press them, instead of rolling out, before you put them on your iron tava to cook.

Devil's advocate

So how can we include an ancient food or eating practice in our daily life?
Nostalgia, like memory, is a funny thing. It can be hyper-focused on one aspect and miss out on the big picture. We can forget how this one detail fitted into the larger scheme of things. Something like that has happened not just with millets but also with all things 'ancient', be it the food – seeds and spices, etc. – or practices like fasting, kriyas and so on. And when we forget how it fits into the larger scheme of things, we reduce it to what it is not – a miracle molecule, or worse, a miracle cure. Then, of course,

the backlash comes that none of this actually works and is all humbug or pseudo-science.

Years ago, I used to do a small session on posture and stretching during Arvind Nadkarni's workshops on communication. He was a brilliant communicator and motivator. This was in the late nineties, when Indian corporate communication had started changing. From hardened sales teams to newly minted CEOs, he would teach them all how to write emails, speak in public and negotiate without breaking into a sweat.

He would swap the traditional U-style conference or classroom seating for gaddas on the floor. I had almost never seen middle-aged men so happy and so eager to learn. I was just starting my career then, and he was a good friend's dad. So he would give me a slot in his one-day or two-day workshops and pay me ₹1,500 for the hour I spoke to his people about health and fitness. I would always look forward to these sessions – opportunity, money, safety, something new to learn and a fun time with Arvind uncle. One of the things I learnt at these sessions was ATTTA – grab their **A**ttention, **T**ell them what you are going to tell them, **T**ell them, **T**ell them what you just told them, and leave them with an **A**ctionable.

Basically, if you have something to say *joh dil ko chu jaaye*, you have to say it right. Similarly, the *tareeka* or method or recipe or process is as critical for the individual ingredients too, to deliver the promise of health and happiness. **And that's why cooking or cuisine is the mainstay**

> of all ancient foods and practices. It teaches you a step-by-step guide to using the ingredient to its full potential, both in terms of taste and efficacy. Culture teaches you how frequently to eat something, celebration or routine, and even guides you as to what to mix it with – ghee, milk, jaggery or rice – based on the occasion. Climate teaches you how to store food and what time of the day to eat it. Essentially, it is difficult to separate culture, climate and cuisine from one another, and without fully utilizing the knowledge of each of them, you stand to only lose from all things ancient.

Food and medicine

Pharmocology is similar to cooking, it's about following the most efficient process/recipe for drug delivery. The paracetamol on your shelf has been made into a round tablet that doesn't hurt the throat when you swallow, has been created with the right delivery agents that the stomach acid can work on, and formulated in the right quantities. If you take too much of paracetamol it could be fatal, too little and there would not even be pain relief.

Essentially, even a routine drug can be ineffective or even dangerous if it's not taken in the right way/context. Lab-made or kitchen-made, without the active ingredients, indications, contra-indications and right dosage, everything is just that – useless at best.

Food combinations, then, matter even more. As we saw, you can't just take millet and make everything out of it. To get the best out of it, you have to take it in the right combos, portions and proportions. Same with seeds or spices. What works are the time-tested processes or recipes. That's why they exist – they are fragile-proof, as they are called. We will learn more about combinations, proportions and portions in the next section of the book.

Section 2

Ghar Ka Khaana Works

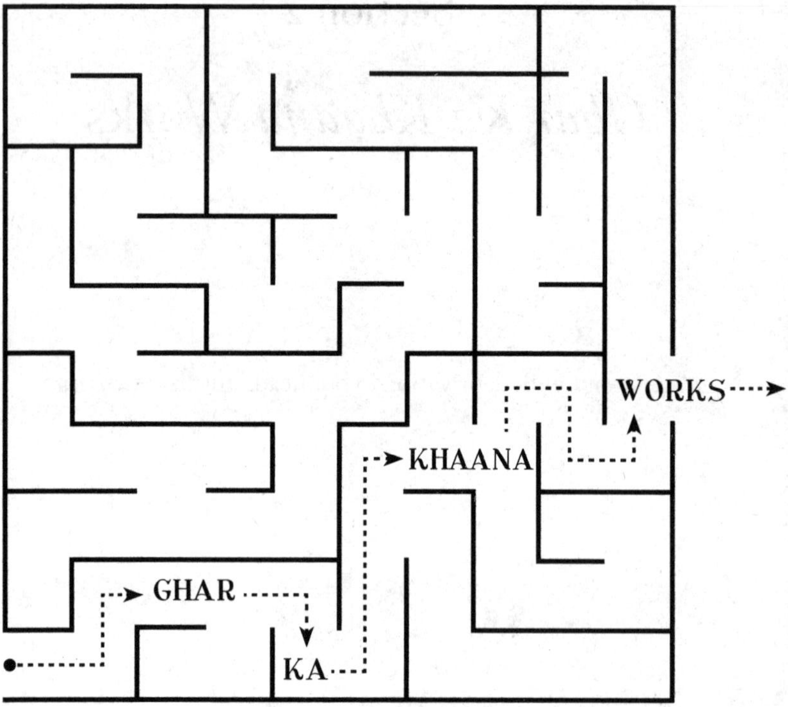

GHAR
KA
KHAANA
WORKS

3

What is a successful diet?

Often when I am working with clients, they say things like, 'This doesn't seem like a diet to me.' This is because diets are synonymous with deprivation in our heads. Just like marriages are with compromise, roads with potholes and work with long hours. So, if we are on a good road we feel as if we are 'abroad', and if we leave the office at 6–7 p.m., we are mocked for having worked a 'half day'. Similarly, if our diet has food that is familiar, inexpensive and delicious, we think that it cannot work. We live in a world where normal is abnormal, unreal, revolutionary almost.

We must, however, normalize the sustainability of diets. The only diet to get on is the one you will keep for life. And that diet is eating *ghar ka khaana*. Quick fixes just don't work. *Sustainability is crucial for success.* It is about shifting slowly, sensitively and steadily towards progress. Whether it is in business with succession planning, or in health with weight-loss goals. Knee-jerk reactions are costly, both in the short and the long term.

Business articles often talk about how an effective leader is someone who can delegate, while a mediocre leader thinks he should save time and do everything himself. One article I read cites the practice of RSVP as an example. The mediocre leader thinks, 'Oh, it's just about one click, let me do it myself.' The visionary leader trains the executive assistant to do it. So it often is a time investment upfront, but in the long term you have saved yourself from a thousand clicks. With weight loss – and health in general – I call upon everyone to be a visionary.

A quick-fix diet that gets you to do a juice for three days, a detox for a week and a cleanse once every couple months, etc., may seem like a good strategy, but keeps you in the loop of dieting for life. I say, save yourself those one thousand RSVP clicks. Liberate yourself with some upfront investment in understanding what exactly you want changed about your body and why, and then build a strategy to get there with sustainable changes to food, exercise and lifestyle.

'Where do you see yourself five years from now?' is the most *faltu* question that anyone can ever ask of a young person when it comes to their work or ambitions. When people ask me that even today, I have no clue what to say. In my career, I couldn't have even dreamt of what life has bestowed me with. Not because I was too scared or timid to dream, but because I was very focused on my day-to-day work. If you keep your head down and your attention on the basics of work, you are able to navigate, upscale and up-skill by default. Though it's a useless question when it comes to your career, it's an important one to answer when it comes to your health and diet.

If five years from now you would like to eat normally and feel confident about wearing anything you feel like without having to worry about a paunch, bra fat and stubby thighs, then you have already signed up for sustainability. If five years from now you see yourself in the latest fasting spa/detox destination, washing up your guilt with *rang berangi* juices, scrolling on your phone to look at pics from five years ago where you looked bloody thin, then you like the diet drama and you can stop reading this book already. Unless, of course, you have had a change of heart, in which case please continue. I also don't want you to stop.

Let me break down what a sustainable (and hence successful) diet means.

a) The diet should not change

No going on or off the diet. That phase doesn't exist. For this to happen the diet must be curated keeping in mind the culture, cuisine and climate you are born into and live in. It must also allow you to connect better with your community, and nothing that you enjoy communally must be in the 'not allowed' or 'avoid' list. Brazil in 2014 and the USA in 2020 put out evidence-backed dietary guidelines for healthy eating. They called upon their populations to eat according to their personal preferences, cultural traditions and budgetary constraints, while avoiding ultra-processed food products (biscuits, chocolates, juices, colas, etc.). Essentially, nutrition science is evolving from its prescriptive model of 'eat x gm of protein, y per cent of fat', etc., towards a commonsensical 'dietary pattern'. A sustainable, sensible and simpler way to eating right and staying healthy.

> ## A dietary pattern
> The quantities, proportions, variety or combination of foods and drinks typically consumed. The dietary pattern approach aims to place emphasis on the total diet as a long-term health determinant instead of focusing on separate foods and nutrients, which may interact with or confound each other.

The prescriptive model is alienating, the dietary pattern is inclusive of all food groups. The prescriptive model confuses people and makes eating a chore. The dietary pattern helps people connect, share and enjoy food, like we were always meant to. Essentially, the dietary pattern is sustainable; you don't count calories, grams, percentages, etc. You do the more basic stuff – choose wholesome, nutritious, fresh food. It has two important aspects:

- Eat more at home
- Eat less out of packets

It really does take as little as that. But sometimes we are averse to simple because we fail to realize that all intelligent designs are simple. Simplicity, as they say, is the ultimate form of sophistication – and I would like to add, of sustainability and success too.

b) The diet should not have levels or phases

One of my clients would often have his sister on his call with our team. The sister would always have her audio on mute and video switched off. It always feels a little weird to be on those kind of calls but we are living in India, and if your client is the only boy in the family after two girls, then you learn to appreciate their need to do so. I have had many such clients. Typically, the boy will listen to everything and nod in agreement, but after the call is done or almost done, the sister will want to question you or bat on behalf of the brother, especially if you have pulled him up over something. This particular sister was very upset after the first call and said to my team that her brother could do better.

Basically, she was telling us to take off those kid gloves and not to give him a diet where he can eat what he wants. 'He's an adult, and he can do what it takes to get in shape,' she said. What she meant was: punish him with a gruelling regime, have him start the day with *bhindi paani*, squeeze juice out of amla and ginger, eat only tempeh or sautéed tofu for dinner, etc. Now, we hate this boy-god situation as much as any sister in the world, but we don't take our revenge through food.

So we explained to her that this is the sustainable diet we want him to be on. We are not giving him a 'basic' diet first – morning, paratha; lunch, dahi–chawal; night, dal–chawal–sabzi, end meal with a banana – only to give him, in the next week, an 'advanced' diet of tempeh, arugula, cauli-rice, ajwain water, etc.

He had been there, done that, and it had left him constipated and cranky. In family dynamics like this, the god experiences the condition but the symptoms are felt by everyone else. If he clears his stomach, his mind will stay calm, he will feel happier, get healthier, and her interventions from Australia could stop. She was on board, and two weeks later, she stopped coming on the calls.

A diet that has phases, where you cleanse first, lean in with fruits later, go on to grilled chicken breast and broccoli or whatever next, is a disaster even before it starts. The first phase and the third or last phase or whatever you call it, have no similarity; they don't even look like books from the same library, forget about looking like pages of the same book.

A sustainable diet attempts to be what it is meant to be till the end of time from day one. Of course, it evolves and adapts to climate – a sherbet in summers instead of a laddoo; to occasions – a cake or a *sheera* as part of a celebratory meal, an extra paratha with friends, and so on. But its true nature stays. Authenticity is important for success.

c) The diet should not be limiting

It should not be limited to just one goal – to lose weight, to reduce HbA1c (by reducing weight), to reduce back pain (by reducing weight) or to fit into that dress (by reducing weight). There is just so much more to life. Our parents are going to die, our children are going to leave us and we are going to see through our spouses. Life is going to give us a lot more to cry about than not fitting into a dress that you could easily get into in 2018.

It's not all going to be gloomy either. A stranger will listen to your life story and change your perspective forever. You are going to get an unexpected upgrade, your song will shoot to the top of the charts, you are going to laugh till you fall at your friend's fortieth, your child will fall in love with you all over again, your partner will order your coffee exactly like you wanted it, you will get clear skies and see a reflection of the Kedar peak in Deoria Tal. A thousand wonderful things, big and small, will happen. The happiness of the scale dropping a few grams, kilos even, or you fitting into a size or two smaller, will fade in comparison.

There are two types of happiness: one that makes you happy every time you think about it, and one that makes you sad every time you think about it. Seeing a smaller number on the scale or fitting into a smaller dress size is the latter kind. Or at least most times it is. For happiness to be long lasting, it must be a consequence of something and not the main thing.

For example, when the happiness is of becoming the CEO, as a natural progression of the path you set yourself on, then it's cool, everlasting. But when 'being the CEO' is the main point, then someone beat you to it early in their career, their take-home is bigger than yours, their wife is skinnier, etc. Weight is like that. So is size. It's just incidental, and inconsequential in the face of everything you will live through and strive for.

Ideal weight

Ideal weight is like the ideal husband – it doesn't exist. But the quest for it does. So, even after working with me since 2008, publishing at least three of my books, my editor said to me:

'This time you must define the right weight. Maybe if I am 55 kg I should not worry much if I get to 60. But should I worry if I get to 80?' I have a hundred ways of answering that, or, rather, questioning that. It will depend on hajaar factors – did you get from 55 to 80 in thirty years or three? Was it the passage of time, a shift of countries, pregnancies, or the consequence of the eight-month bed rest you had after that terrible road accident? Questions are many, and the answer is not in body weight.

'There is no such thing as a good husband,' Anupam Kher said to me. His niece was about to get married and I had just asked him, 'How's the guy?' and he was a bit emotional. 'I told my niece, "Good-looking *nahi*, kind husband *dhoondo*." Waise, why do girls even need to get married these days? My niece can do everything on her own; in that sense she doesn't need a man or marriage, but kindness, Rujuta ji, we all need. I will never think that any man is good for my niece, but if she finds a kind man, someone who gets her point, is respectful of what she wants out of life, is not possessive, then that's all. *Toh haan*, the boy is kind. He understands her,' he said with sincerity.

> So the answer to what is ideal weight is just this – **it should be weight that is kind to your body**. Doesn't get in your way, doesn't load your joints, doesn't throw off your blood sugars or blood pressure. *Bas. Baaki,* your body is more than capable of handling life on its own.

In June 2023, the American Medical Association (AMA) updated its guidelines,[7] asking primary-care physicians to make assessments of people based on not just their body weight (or BMI) but by looking at other factors, too. So far, the BMI that was believed to be ideal wasn't a fair representation of ethnicity, gender, age, etc., and therefore an imperfect clinical measure. The new guideline asked them to factor in the waist-to-hip ratio, visceral fat, exercise frequency, etc., before making assessments of health. The latest research presented in *The Lancet* journal in January 2025 also revised the definition of being overweight or obese, moving beyond body weight/BMI to now including more parameters like waist measurement, musculature, etc.

This is a chart I had made during the lockdown to highlight the differences between sustainable and unsustainable diets. I think you will find it useful.

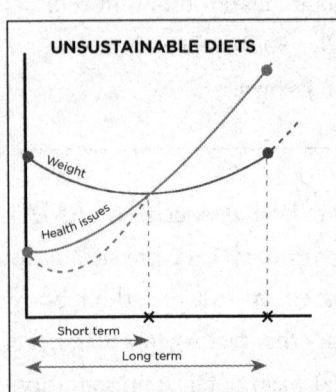

UNSUSTAINABLE DIETS

- In the short term, you lose weight, but at the cost of health.
- Due to the placebo effect, you may mistakenly believe that health is improving.
- In the long term, the weight comes back, and this time with many more health issues.

- Focus on carbs/proteins/fats/calories.
- Deprivation of food groups or calories.
- Examples – Keto, LCHF, Paleo, IF, Atkins, etc. Always comes with a name
- Arbitrary rules – skip meals, eat non-traditional meals, calorie deficit, compensation diet, count macros.

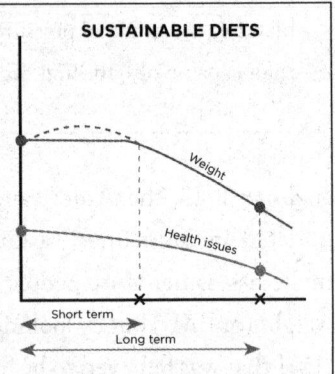

SUSTAINABLE DIETS

- In the short term, you might not see a weight loss, but health starts to improve.
- In fact, there could be an increase in total weight, due to increase in lean body weight.
- In the long term, weight reduces and health improves consistently and irreversibly.

- Focus on local/seasonal/traditional.
- No deprivation, intuitive eating.
- Examples – home-cooked food, seasonal specialties, traditional cooking methods.
- Commonsense rules – no long meal gaps, eat slowly and without distractions, time-tested meal combos and proportions.

4

The real meaning of *ghar ka khaana*

Nutrition science started as a field to understand, intervene in and prevent malnourishment. More specifically, to stop the deformity and deaths that lack of nutrients produced. At least, that was its primary function. 'Post industrialization, it changed a bit, and today it seems to have entirely played into the hands of the food industry,' said a professor of biochemistry at a nutrition conference I was attending, back in 2012. 'First they sold us readymade bread, then they put the fibre back in the dough and marked it up by 20 per cent, and now it's the era of the gluten-free bread at a 40 per cent mark up.'

Nutrition science was always meant to be a public health service. When it moves away from that goal, science becomes sciency. But when it doesn't, then it discovers over and over again that food isn't just molecules. That eventually nutrition science is not complete without looking at climate, cuisine, culture, crop cycle. That food is also a language of love, politics and even religion. That it is also about gender, economics and survival.

Today, as we saw in the last chapter, food or nutrition science is firmly establishing itself in your grandmom's philosophy of eating and living well. So, more than food groups, calories or portion control, dietary guidelines are establishing themselves in dietary patterns, i.e., the general eating habits or the food customs of a community or a region, etc. In short, *ghar ka khaana*.

> ## *Ghar ka khaana*
> Food cooked at home, using ingredients that grow in a field around you (*local*), incorporating *seasonal* produce and using time-tested recipes and techniques (*traditional*).

The 80:20 ratio is an important rule of thumb and is applicable in many aspects of life. It's a useful tool for identifying the most important factors and focusing on them to improve results. Applied to business, it says that 80 per cent of your income will come from 20 per cent of your products, clients, services, etc. Applied to food, it means that to maintain good health, *80 per cent of what you eat must be ghar ka khaana* – food that is cooked in your kitchen and is consumed with, to borrow from Insta lingo, an attitude of gratitude. Local. Seasonal. Traditional. It is as simple as that.

What's local?

In my first book, I had written how Shimla Baba had left me underwhelmed with his rather simple answer. I had met him in 2004 and had asked him, 'Who brought you here?'

He replied, 'The same one who brought you here.' This was in his cave in Tapovan, high above Gaumukh. '*Dhongi saala*,' I thought to myself, only to realize years later that what he had said was the opposite of fake. It was the hard truth. It took me years to realize that simplicity is profound.

In 2022, I went on a much less demanding hike along the Prachin Badrinath *paidal marg*, the ancient trade and pilgrimage route to Badrinath from Rishikesh. On a bend along the river (opposite Taj Rishikesh), lives a baba. He has been there for years, and no one knows exactly when he came and where he is from. So when my guide and I stopped by at the *kutir*, I asked him, '*Aap kaha se ho?*'

My question seemed to have irked him. '*Kya matlab?*' he barked. '*Jaha ho, wahi ke ho.*' (Wherever you are now is where you belong.) My only growth from 2004 to 2022 was that I got that funda instantly. I was looking for an internet connection to check on my dad who wasn't keeping too well. That reality check was all I needed to put my phone back. You can't micromanage from a distance; you can either trek or be by the bedside. I had already made my choice.

Eating local means just that – eat according to where you are physically now. Don't let your screen transport you into eating or drinking some novel, expensive food that featured in your favourite celeb's 'What I eat in a day' reel. Keep things real and grounded. Kanji over kombucha, rice over quinoa, mango over blueberries.

The importance of local

Eating local is crucial for the health of the people and the planet. I think everyone understands that. But eating local is important for communities too. There is no chance of connecting, loving and accepting each other without sharing our *sukh–dukh* over food. The only time you can share is if you have something to offer, whether it's gossip or food. I am sure there's some study somewhere that says that people who share gossip and food are more intelligent or successful, or that it is linked to our evolution or it is what separates us, *Homo sapiens*, from the rest of the animal kingdom. Our ability to laugh, grieve, love and connect over food.

One of my share market clients – sharp as a knife she is – often tells me that the equity market is not risky but the increasing longevity and the loneliness it can potentially bring is. You may have enough to eat, but who will you share it with? One of the biggest things that dieting takes away from us is the ability to eat freely, and therefore share fearlessly and live fully.

IMHO, the reason why we live in a polarized world today is because we are all caught in the web of grabbing more protein per calorie, avoiding sugar at all costs and sneaking in more avocado for good fat. Our ability to appreciate each other's food, and therefore POV, is gone. Looked down upon even. We only eat with those who eat like us – at 2 p.m., or clean, or keto.

The echo chamber depletes us of our energy, not body fat. Local food, hearty laughter, disagreements that don't last beyond a day, are the need of the hour. *Lassi aur ladai jitni badhao utni badh sakti hai.* Give me an equivalent of wisdom, reciprocation and de-escalation with broccoli or Greek yoghurt.

Local means inclusivity. It means not reducing food to its nutrients (Michael Pollan calls it nutritionism, like ageism, sexism, racism, etc.) but celebrating it for all its glory. One of the easy ways to decide what is local to you is to check if it has a name in your mother tongue or in the regional language. This is a crucial test.

A name in the local language means that not just you, but also the bees, the butterflies and the birds of the region recognize it as food. Embracing local means embracing our identity, our uniqueness, our differences. And empowering our diets with the crucial ingredient that diets rob us of – diversity. Diverse diets are the need of the hour. Nutrition science knows that diverse diets that are in sync with the culture, climate and crop cycles are the best carriers of all nutrients. All nutrients, including the ones considered to be scarce, like protein, folic acid or magnesium.

But it takes a certain amount of scientific temper and distance from social media to understand this truth. Or else we just spend our time hopping from one diet to another, moving far away from *ghar ka khaana*. Local food, home food, nurturing food becomes the enemy in the name of science. If there is a definition of irony, this is it.

Boston–Bangkok–Bangalore

I had written in 2009 about how quinoa, the latest superfood, is not something you needed to be on and how dal-chawal could serve you just as well. It's 2024, quinoa is still around and one of my clients' mom had just taken cooking classes and made a quinoa–raspberry salad. My young client had relished it, but I had marked it in red on her weekly recall sheet. She wanted to know why. 'Why is it in red – it's healthy, right? Fibre and veg protein.'

'Fibre and veg protein ke hundred options you have in your diet.'

'But then, what's the problem with quinoa?' she asked. So I told her about the *Boston–Bangkok–Bangalore formula*. If something is available across all cities globally, is known by the same name and for the same nutrients, don't eat it. Rucola, arugula, avocado, chia, almond milk, olive oil – all fall in the same category.

When the rich across the globe obsess over the same food, it means change of land usage for the poor. Quinoa, for example, is the food of native South American people. But now, with the global rich wanting it, a lot of their land that is under cultivation has to be dedicated to quinoa, often at the cost of rotating crops and growing diverse species. Then there's also predatory pricing, where farmers are forced to sell the crop to middlemen and at a price they fix, much like drug cartels. Fibre for one, fear for another.

Same with chocolates. On the Ivory Coast, for example, the cocoa trees are being planted by burning down old forests. Then there is the ethical issue of children being employed to pick the cocoa, often at the cost of school and education. All this to keep the price at a certain point and profits at another.

We are all children of the same earth, our resources are shared. That is what *vasudhaiva kutumbakam* means. Take only what is needed and live within your ecological means. So, my young client, who studied in Tufts and lives in Kolkata, doesn't have to give up on quinoa, she only needs to recognize it as fancy food and not eat it solely for nutrients. But she can eat it as a fancy food, something you eat to show off, or as an occasional indulgence. Regulated to once a month max. Same with avocado toast, dark chocolate, chia pudding, etc., ok? Now breathe.

How Anushree stopped fighting with her mom

Anushree Reddy, the trailblazing designer, is one of my clients. Sitting in my office, sipping on kokum sherbet, she said to me in her Hyderabadi accent, 'Rujuta, I was so scared at first. Idli in the morning, rice for lunch, palli (peanuts) with coffee and some more rice for dinner. I was not eating any carbs earlier and still I was not losing any weight, and then I thought so much carbs, what will happen now? And now I am losing weight, inches, my cravings are down, my parents are happy, you know.

'Earlier my mother would call and ask, "What will you eat for Sunday lunch?" Once I would go there, we would be fighting because I wouldn't touch anything she had cooked. My dad was just so fed up. Now I tell them, make whatever you want, and I am eating, enjoying.

I am not a client-facing designer, full time I am working at the factory. You know how that is – it's a mess. And full of stress. Everyone is screaming. But now I am screaming less. And right now, when all of Hyderabad is down with chikungunya, I am slogging at the factory and nothing, nothing has happened to me. First when I was on low carb, no carb, weight I am not losing, but the first infection person in Hyderabad is me.'

'Oh! Anushree, I want to quote you in my book,' I said.

'Ya, ya please, with my full name and details please.'

So go and buy her great stuff from Linking road, Khar, right next to my office.

What's seasonal?

In India we recognize six specific seasons and six specific tastes – Vasanta, Grishma, Varsha, Sharata, Hemanta and Shishira (Spring, Summer, Rains, Autumn, Pre-winter and Winter) are the seasons. Madhura, Tikhta, Kashaya, Katu, Amla and Lavana (sweet, bitter, astringent, pungent, sour and salty) are the tastes. The seasons are called *ritu*s and tastes are *rasa*s in Sanskrit. The belief is that you need to nurture all tastes in your life to enjoy good health and relish every season.

When people go on diets, it's the seasonal variations that get hit. Invariably, your mojo, moods and immunity sinks. This happens at both ends of the sciency and satvik spectrum. Deprivation, monotony and boredom is the bottom line and there's almost no room left for sunshine, rain or snow.

Bharatiya sanskriti isn't just about celebrating the diversity of the seasons with different foods, but also with different parts of the same plant based on the season. So there will be tender *haldi achaar* with lemon in the spring, a haldi-dominant sweet with ghee in the winters (*adadhiyo*) and a haldi-leaf-wrapped coconut-and-rice delicacy for you to savour in the rains (*patoli*). Quite different from the *haldi paani* or the curcumin pill for immunity and eye health.

Or turning carrots into *kali gajar kanji*, fresh carrot achaar and gajar halwa – a pungent, tangy and sweet way to welcome winter. We have traded this for the daily dose of ABC juice. This is like turning ₹1 lakh into ₹12,000 – *laakh na baar hajaar kari deedha*, which is an old Gujarati saying for settling for something much lesser because of your inability to see the value in what you already have. (Turn to page 216 to see a table of foods illustrating this point).

The neem flower is a sherbet of the spring, its leaves ka chutney a *prasad* on Gudi Padwa (the new year for many regions in India) and the bitter-sweet fruit, nimbuli, a treat that kids in Pind of Punjab would look forward to. The millets too are consumed as per the season, as we discovered in the previous section.

You get my drift, right? Kalidasa wrote about ritus, Gulzar sahab composed couplets about them, your grandmom cooked according to it, but you have sold your soul and *dimaag* to viral trends. Well done. ₹1 lakh to ₹12,000. It's just like what @aiyoshraddha says – you need many mornings in one day, because you need to take moringa powder, an amla shot, *haldi paani*, apple cider vinegar, etc.

The intelligence that you may find the neem leaves bitter but won't mind its fruit or prefer its sherbet is gone with the wind. And the wind is polluted. Because when cultures lose cuisine, the crop cycle is challenged. Land use changes, and only cash crops that fit the BBB formula get prominence, at the cost of local fare. That's how we are losing the seasonal delicacies of our regions. Or else we would be sipping on *kulith kalan* in summers in Goa and eating a *gehat paratha* in the winters in Rishikesh.

Now, regardless of when and where you holiday, it is the same two-minute noodles by the roadside and the same almond milk latte in posh cafes. Seasonal food practices and rituals were intact and in place until just about thirty years ago. The late nineties came with economic reforms and liberalization, and it helped us to get where we are now. We are better off today, yes, but we didn't fully anticipate the cuisine losses that it would bring.

What's traditional

In its simplest form, it means cooking food at home using time-tested recipes. The highlight of traditional food is that it is diverse and requires eating in set combinations. It puts to good use all the ingredients that are available in the season and the region, and uses culinary art and wisdom to turn them into meals that are both delicious and nutritious. The combinations differ, based on whether you are celebrating, grieving or simply having a regular day. **Food is used as a medium that acts as an interface between you and your circumstances**. It is used to temper sadness, enhance happiness and embrace the vagueness of a routine life

Eating traditional food has one constraint though – most of it is taught orally. It is handed down over generations and its context/greatness, like love, is hidden in plain sight. But we are fast losing not just languages but also the nuances of it. 'When was the last time someone spoke to you in a *muhawara*?' asked Javed Akhtar at a literary event recently.

When skill and sophistication with language are lost, it has an impact on our kitchens too. The special dishes cooked on certain days are now forgotten, and their recipes are hard to come by. Everything of value is now said only in English, and we live in a world where traditional either signals exotic or backward. Loss of languages has meant loss of fluency and ease in our eating and living.

But isn't traditional food fattening?

People genuinely believe that we no longer have the luxury of eating food in a commonsensical or uncomplicated manner because we are no longer burning the calories we used to. This, in fact, is the most widely used argument against local, seasonal and traditional food – that unlike our ancestors, we are not active enough. We are not walking around, foraging, hunting, or even cleaning, sweeping and washing the way we used to before. And since we don't live like them, we cannot eat like them.

However, scientific experiments using the doubly labelled water method – the gold standard to measure calories burned daily in normal life (energy expenditure) – have, proved that sedentary city dwellers in the West, traditional farmers in South America and hunter-gatherers in Africa pretty much burn the same calories per day.

But we are so taken in by the 'move-more-burn-more' dogma that we don't stop to think if it stands the test of empirical data, critical thinking or experimental evidence. By the way, even animals in labs or zoos have the same daily calorie expenditure as those in the wild. In fact, when differences in individuals are measured, couch potatoes burn only about 200 calories less than people who make it a point to exercise and stay active. So yes, all those videos that told you that if you eat first at a *shaadi* and then dance, it burns the calories, are lies. As are viral tweets that blame 'Indian food' for the obesity epidemic.

As humans, we evolved uniquely, developing traits that required a lot of calories[8] (also known as the basal metabolic rate [BMR]), just to keep functioning. And our cooking, or cuisine, evolved as a sophisticated, clever way to provide the body – and especially the brain – with the calories it needs. Not just to survive but to thrive. Metabolism is much more complex than calories in and out, or whatever else that it has been reduced to.

Don't count

One of my clients is a young boy in his twenties, just back from studies and already in daddy's retail business. A fat teen, he worked very hard to lose weight when he was studying in Dublin. But now that he was back, he was having a hard time keeping it off. 'I try and keep my calories low,' he told me. 'I calculate return on calories, so steak is the best and fries are the worst,' he continued. He had returned during the shraadh period. 'So yesterday it was grandpa *ka shraadh*. My bua lives very close, and today she asked me to come over. It was her grandmother-in-law ka shraadh and she's just passed away last year and I wasn't there. In fifteen days, I have had four shraadh meals.' (These tend to be big meals with poori, kheer, etc., and the belief is that everything must be eaten and nothing left on the plate.)

'Ah! Very Indian problems you are having,' I said to him. He was a single child but from a big joint family. 'I am sure you will take your dad's business places, but what will enrich your life is connecting to your culture, community and even climate. And food is a good place to start. You understand these valuable Cs and it will help you with the R.'

'Returns?' he asked.

'Retail,' I replied.

'But RD, *calories toh calories hai na?*'

'Yes, but not at the cost of overlooking culture, climate, cuisine, community. Both steak and fries are useless on these parameters.'

'So don't eat both?'

'Eat them. But occasionally, and don't sweat the shraadh, Dussera, Diwali meals. If you must use calories as a measure, use the other Cs too.'

He had studied Operations Research (using mathematics to optimize processes), so we decided that all these Cs would get equal weightage.

'Sounds good.'

I would like calories out of the picture entirely, but I am mature, so I count a win when I have one. The next time

> around when he ate, he would not make the mistake of only counting numbers. Or looking at the merits/demerits of anything on just one data point.
>
> We even added more Cs to food over time. So if he asked for a meeting, he just eats whatever his client or supplier is eating – *connection*. Good for business. If a store has done exceptional business and the store manager calls for samosa and jalebi – eat with everyone. *Celebration*. Good for business. If you know a tough customer likes Mysore paak, carry it and offer it and eat it – and gain some personal *credit*. Good for business. You wanna *patao* a girl, eat what she's eating – *chivalry*, good for the business of life. Long story short, live your life outside the box of calories.

We don't need to shift away from traditional diets, but we need policy intervention to fix the obesogenic environment we live in – the unchecked penetration of junk food, the unwalkable cities and towns, the polluted air, depletion of green spaces, the list really is endless.

5

The three rules of eating
ghar ka khaana

Like all languages, *ghar ka khaana* has its own grammar and rules. These rules aren't written in stone; they evolve with time, but you must understand them to appreciate them. They are more like a framework, and within that framework you are free to do as you please. If you have learnt a classical art form – dance, singing or playing an instrument – then you know what I mean. These frameworks are in place like a safety guard, to ensure that you don't hurt yourself or anyone else in the process.

Similarly, the rules of *ghar ka khaana* ensure that your eating has depth. That it is not merely an act of consumption but *there is adequate attention to digestion, absorption, assimilation and excretion.*

When these rules are followed, the entire body feels rejuvenated and refreshed. You spend less time thinking and strategizing how to optimize protein or anything else and more time enjoying and living life. These rules work in the background, and eating right becomes a set pattern, a default. It ensures that without needing to constantly calculate, you eat right.

Now, spelling out food rules is a bit like explaining how the rose smells. But my editor refuses to publish the book without it, so this is me trying my best to give you some guidelines to work with. They come with a disclaimer – that you will truly understand and appreciate them only after a lifetime of practice. There's a reason why the old works, because it is fresh every time you encounter it, like a hot cup of chai.

So here are the three food rules or three ways in which *ghar ka khaana* works.

Rule 1: Eat in the right combinations

The greatness of *ghar ka khaana* comes from the combinations we eat it in. It's teamwork. You can think of *food combinations as mangroves that prevent you from getting swept away by trends and viral videos.* These combos ensure that active ingredients of food are delivered with love and care, and in commonsense ways that have stood the test of time.

Let's look at a few examples (some we have come across in the book earlier).

Haldi may have curcumin and it may have anti-inflammatory properties, but it works best when consumed in combinations like the *haldi-doodh* when you are feeling a bit low, in the tadka as a routine practice, the *haldi sabzi and roti* in the winters, and so on.

Millets today may have the recognition because they got the government's push, but for them to be truly as nutritious as they can be, their combinations must be respected. A thumb rule for all millets is that they must be mixed with dairy fat – milk, makhan or ghee. In the absence of these, millets are heavy to digest. They are also routinely eaten with chutneys like peanut, til, flaxseed, garlic, etc., an infusion of seeds and spices to ease digestion.

There is another unwritten rule – that when you turn them into laddoos or barfi, you always use jaggery, and not sugar. Bajra has this rule that even if you just eat a *rotla* or a bhakri, you must eat or finish the meal with a piece of jaggery.

Similarly, there are rules for mixing grains and pulses too. I remember, a long time ago, before gluten was a thing, there was a food festival at Carter Road. I went to the SNDT University (my alma mater) food stall. The girls there had made rajma paratha. 'What's that?' I wondered. 'Boil the rajma, mash it, pack it inside the wheat atta like aloo, and voila, rajma paratha is ready.'

I know how you are taught to think in nutrition schools. You have to somehow increase the protein content of a food by making combinations that never even existed, like rajma paratha. You do some random calculations on paper, and there it is. You never have to think of digestibility or useability; for how long this paratha stays palatable, let alone tasty, after it is made. Food on paper is different from food in the pet or inside the stomach.

The three rules of eating *ghar ka khaana*

Actually, we should be taught how to increase protein digestibility in foods like rajma–chawal, a combination that has always existed. It is easy to digest and a delicacy for lazy Sunday afternoons. You can even reheat rajma and eat it with another batch of rice. And you can add a *boondi raita* or a *chaas* or plain dahi for improved protein, etc.

But we are trained from the nutrient aspect, without keeping the end user or design viability in the picture. Because in real life, outside of the lab, when you tell your client to have a glass of chaas with the rajma–chawal, he's burping and farting less and feeling lighter. And recommending you to his friends and family for easy tips that got him thin. This is also how you make money.

But to be honest, rajma–chawal with raita or chaas is also a combination that has always existed. So you can't really learn anything new in a nutrition school, but you can learn the value and the practicality of old foods. You can learn why time-tested combos work even in present times. You can design experiments that have you checking on people for at least twenty-four hours, post their consumption of your recommended meal and not just calculate protein or calories on paper and then score marks for the most protein in lowest calorific value. We can be real and learn 'most protein with least farts in 24 hours', but that's a topic and a rant for another day.

So the thumb rule here is that the big pulses – like rajma and chana – are mixed with rice, and the smaller ones – like lobia, moong and matki – have the flexibility to go with rice, roti or millets.

Peas and meat alternatives

When I started working, people on diets would avoid peas because they were thought of as fattening. Just like they would avoid ghee or rice and have sukha roti instead. But now roti is gluten, and hence bad. Rice was once just starch and hence bad, but now it is resistant starch, a prebiotic, hence good. Ghee was fat, hence bad. Now it's short-chain fatty acids, fat-burning, hence good. Same with peas.

First, they were high-calorie, hence bad. Now they are vegan protein, hence good. '*Ab, yeh last village nahi ma'am, first village hai,*' my driver Chinu said about Mana, the last village after Badrinath.

'*Yeh, kab hua?*'

'*PM visit ke baad,*' he said. Rebranding is not just in dieting.

The backlash to excessive consumption of meat has been to look for more kind, sustainable sources of protein. But what we got instead is the same companies that sell us dairy and meat, selling us almond milk, mock meat, 3D-printed lamb, etc. Eating animal protein is not unsustainable when done in time-tested portions, proportions and frequency (more on that later). And eating non-dairy, alternative meats that are highly processed isn't the answer either.

Rule 2: Eat food in the right proportions

The proportion of every ingredient in the kitchen is pre-fixed. Inclusivity at its best – ensuring that no one ingredient gets to dominate the food plate at the cost of the other.

Some proportions are very obvious, and we all know them – for khichdi it is 3:1 of rice and moong dal, for idli 2.5:1 and for dosa 3:1 of rice and urad dal. This is how you would get light meals, food that leaves you satiated, that allows you to sleep well, wake up in the morning and exercise. The protein fixation has changed this to about 2:1 in recent times, but the thumb rule – that grains or millets should be in a significantly higher ratio than pulses or legumes – stays.

Eating in the right proportion would mean that your meal/thali will have grains or millets, along with the legumes or dals, and then a cooked sabzi that is almost the same proportion as dal (or slightly lesser). The accompaniments – like the salad, chutney, achar or raita – together cannot be more than the amount of the cooked sabzi. This makes for a complete meal (check the chart on page 150). One that is gentle on your stomach, bandwidth and pocket. A meal that gives you not just fibre, protein, fat and magnesium, but also your vitamin B and C, zinc, anthocyanins, etc.

Your favourite keto or protein diet proponent asking you to take 30 grams of fibre and 30 grams of fat along with 30 grams of protein is a poorer version of these time-tested proportions. ₹1 lakh to ₹12,000.

The timeless method of proportions doesn't just lend itself to being positioned as wholesome. In fact, it makes for the very definition of boring/gharelu food. But just as love bombing is a red flag, protein bombing or good-bacteria bombing is a red flag too. Green flags in relationships are more like texts that that read – done, cool, send OTP. **Routine love and meals are very boring**. They have the chemistry but not the volatility.

Proportions, combinations, seasons keep interacting with each other all the time to create diversity in all traditional diets. Like jowar is a millet of the summers, but in parts of Maharashtra, it is used in the 3:1 proportion with black urad dal along with one teaspoon of methi seeds to create the bhakri of the winters.

The Himalayan region has a similar ritual of making *gehat paratha* – made with horse gram and wheat atta – to stay warm at the peak of winter. So-called 'heaty' and 'cooling' foods are mixed in pre-set proportions to add diversity to cooking and optimize nutrient delivery in the most delicious ways.

A Gujarati client of mine had grown up in Sudan and had married in Ahmedabad. She would make a delicious aam pickle with chana in it – a legacy of the land she grew up in. Intelligent use of resources (local and seasonal produce) in the kitchen is one of the most creative ways to make diets healthy, affordable and accessible.

New age health influencers don't get this. They are filled with rigid ideas of what makes for heaty or cooling foods. No course, however long, can teach you everything you need to learn. Which is why in real life, whether your qualification is for seven years, months or days, you must learn to listen. You must adapt and respect living traditions and appreciate the tweaks they come with.

From millets to grains, from legumes to pulses, from wild vegetables to the ones cultivated, from nuts to seeds, from spices to herbs, from wild fruits to those carefully nurtured, from milk to meat, the Indian kitchen has proportions in which all these are eaten. Through meals that gently remind us that we are just a part of the whole. Food, in India, is not medicine for a disease but a reflection of the divinity that lies within each one of us. If diversity, inclusivity and oneness had a name, it would be *dal-chawal-ghee*.

Pee halad aani ho gori (Drink a lot of haldi and turn fair overnight) is a Marathi idiom reeking of sarcasm and mocks the gullible who use large doses of a food product to fix something. It is a not-so-gentle reminder that the power of food can only be harnessed optimally with unwritten kitchen rules, the most important of which is proportion. Everything in the right amount heals, and too much hurts. Even if it's just *paani aur pyaar*.

The Saif way to eat meat

One of the things that is strictly proportioned in the classical Indian diet is meat. Travel to the remote Himalaya and you will see how a whole village will share a goat or even a yak. Closer home, Maharashtra is probably most serious about the proportion in which meat, fish and even eggs will be consumed. Through the month of Shravan, according to the lunar calendar, there's complete abstinence from meat, fish and even eggs. It compulsorily makes room for neglected vegetables, dals and even nuts, and brings about a refreshing change to the monotony in the kitchen. In fact, even on a regular basis, non-veg which also includes egg in the Indian context) is limited to just a few days of the week, mostly Wednesdays, Fridays and Sundays.

These are climate-resilient practices. Sustainability is ingrained in our DNA; it breathes through our culture and cuisine. Recently, the World Wildlife Fund declared that Indian diets are the most climate-friendly and sustainable, exactly for this reason. Even in parts of India where there are no such observances with meat (like in Maharashtra), it is consumed only as a part of the whole meal. It doesn't mean taking millets, rice, veggies, fruits and nuts, etc., off the plate. It simply exists along with everyone else.

Saif, who loves his holidays (he's the OG work–life balance ambassador) – UK in summers, Gstaad in winters – has an eating formula. He is predominantly vegetarian when at home in Mumbai and dominantly non-vegetarian when abroad. 'Because where else can you get the parwal, lauki, bhindi, turai, palak, chavli, etc.? And no one can make a great fish and chips or roast at home.'

'But my doctor says'

A client of mine was a politician. He was obese and desperate to lose weight. Late nights, skipped meals, large meals, stress, alcohol, smoking were all a part of his routine and some were occupational hazards. His lipid profile was a bit off, within range but at the higher end. He would eat only egg whites for breakfast, and I recommended that he have two whole eggs with a buttered toast when travelling, and chapati when at home.

'Kaun hai yeh pagal dietitian?' His doctor demanded to know after he heard that six egg whites were replaced with two whole eggs and chapati or toast. 'Will she take responsibility for your heart attack after all that yolk chokes your arteries?' Earlier in my career, some doctors have called me on the landline to fire me for asking their clients to eat ghee, rice, coconut, etc. They have demanded to know if I was out of my mind or have ever had my brain checked. One even offered to do it for free.

But apne ko thappad se nahi, pyar se dar lagta hai.

'Then what did he say?' I asked my client.

'After I said that I am now actually eating less at breakfast [earlier, after egg whites, he would eat one glucose biscuit ka packet and one glass of orange juice, freshly squeezed], my legs are not hurting in the night and am generally feeling light, the doctor got even more angry. He told me that the main thing was to lose weight, so just eat 1 kg of fruit for breakfast and you will lose 10 kgs in a month. He has even allowed me any choice of fruits in the morning. 'Any time you will drop dead with this weight,' the doctor had declared. 'Will your dietitian come to save you?'

'No problem, *karo aap*,' I said to him (at least it wasn't advice to skip breakfast entirely). I have always been quite clear that clients who are already hassled with their health should not be bothered further. One kilogram of fruit in one day, and in just one meal, makes no sense. It would mean risking higher triglycerides levels over time, but I knew better than to say that to my client when he was already in the grip of fear. 'If you find yourself eating glucose biscuits, aching legs and poor sleep again, go back to eating like you were in the last three months' was the only advice I offered. That was our last meeting. I have learnt that you must honour your clients' trust in you to tell you things as they are and leave in a way that they are not intimidated or embarrassed if they have to approach you again.

The overreach of doctors and the under-reach of common sense while making food decisions continues to remain a high barrier for sustainable diets and fitness.

Rule 3: Eat the right portions

So much is spoken about longevity these days, but in the noise we often forget that life is unpredictable and that eating with pleasure is a rare joy. We have made eating a painful activity, one where we are either second-guessing whether or not to go for the next bite or are rushing through it while scrolling through our feeds.

We are all scared of age and death. Almost everything we do in life, including the pursuit to lose weight or get fit, is an escape from this reality. But when reality hits us, we realize that we lose appetite with age and eventually a dead body cannot consume anything at all. We are here for a limited time, and while we are here we must make the most of our primal joy of food. Use it as a fuel to pursue all that we see meaning in.

My partner runs Connect with Himalaya and wrote a book on his Himalayan travels and its people and the culture. Much to his delight, he received an email from Bill Aitken, praising the book. One of our big moments for sure. Bill Aitken is Scottish, hitchhiked to India in 1959, fell in love with the Himalaya and an Indian princess, stayed back in the mountains and made Mussoorie his home. Along the way he wrote some of the best books on the Himalaya and India. In 2014, we visited him to thank him for his grand gesture and struck a friendship.

Every time we are around Mussoorie, GP tells me we must visit him – 'Don't know how many good years he has left.' At one such meeting I said to Bill, 'One time, let us take you out to lunch instead of eating at your home.'

'Good food,' he asked?

'Promise,' I said. I took both the boys to Padmini Niwas on the Mall Road. Gujju thali is their specialty, but they are always kind enough to accommodate my request and make a few local delicacies too.

So there we were eating lunch – *mandua roti, gehat-stuffed poori, chainsu, palak kafli, Kumaoni raita, red rice, Gujarati dal, mooli thechwani, jhangora kheer*. And a special item – aloo–tamatar shaak. We ate and exchanged stories of bike rides, mystics, treks, and shepherds that appear and disappear into the fog. Where there is warmth, love and connection, the stomach dilates, the appetite is roused and everything is tastier and even lighter.

But a lot more than the conversation, I was much taken by Bill's appetite. He ate everything on the plate and then asked for a second helping of jhangora kheer. Men with a robust appetite, who can eat with delight, are a turn-on for me. Not that this was a competition, but GP hadn't eaten half of what Bill had, and I had eaten only half of what GP had.

'Hum log iske pehle tapkenge,' I told GP. 'Your mountain man is going nowhere.' Later, Bill walked swiftly up the Mall Road. 'Ah, it was a good meal,' he said to me.

'Ah, you are a good man,' I said to him.

The brave and the creative have a voracious appetite for life. And it will reflect in their relationship with food too. Because what is food if not life?

But how does one not overeat?

It takes time and even a leap of self-discovery, but you have to begin by trusting your ability to self-terminate the act of eating. We are all born with it but lose it to grabbing lunches, sending emails over breakfast and Netflixing dinners. And then of course, we just don't eat wholesome food because we are so scared of home food.

The whole point is that if food is flavourful and nurtures all the six tastes, then you are likely to eat just the right quantities. Or to put it in another way – a lot less than what you fear you will eat if food is delicious. And every time you try 'tricking' your stomach – by first having salad, then some protein, and lastly some carbs – you are going to open the fridge later looking for some low-volume, high-density, poor-nourishment calories. So you consume fewer calories at meal time only to overeat closer to your bedtime. Your ring is not going to be happy with you the next day.

Dr Badwe is known as 'dev manus', or God-figure, in Mumbai, thanks to his compassionate and caring work at Tata Memorial Hospital. We were together on a podcast for Tata trust on breast cancer awareness. He was talking about preventive measures – self-examination being one of them – and I was talking about food. During our chat he said we must realize that *there is a thin line between vigilance and anxiety*. By all means be vigilant about your breasts, about your health, but don't be anxious. First learn what a normal breast feels like in every phase of your menstrual cycle, because otherwise everything is going to feel like a lump and that's not helpful at all. I wanted to stand up and applaud.

The thing about people with a solid practice is that they make the complex easy, within reach of all of us to grasp. So when it comes to portions too, be vigilant and not anxious. And just like how the breast will look and feel different depending on the phase of your menstrual cycle, the appetite will differ too. The changes are mild, but if you lose track of your normal appetite, you will always feel like you are eating too much. So you go about most of your days under-eating, only to overeat a cheesecake, a chocolate pastry and a tub of ice-cream during PMS. Remember that high variance, whether in a performance or a person, in pleasure or pain, breast or bhukh, should get flagged.

The Jordan formula

If you still need more clues on how much to eat, then try the Jordan formula. I was in Amman for a YPO talk, and I learnt of a beautiful Arabic tradition. Your host will welcome you with Arabic coffee and dates, and you take one of each. Your host will goad you to have another one; *manvar*, *agrah*, indulging you with food, nudging you to eat just a little more, is a part of every culture. An exchange of warmth and love. But in the Arabic tradition, you must refuse the second date and coffee if you think you cannot have the third one. This, I feel, is such a beautiful way to relish what one eats and

> not overdo it. And the framework is open – have the second one if you can also have the third one. The fourth one if you can have the fifth. But if you can't, stop at the odd number, don't go even.

Mental Meal Map

When the eyes become clear, the body healthy and the appetite increases, it's a sign of success, according to the *Hatha Yoga Pradipika*. No wonder, then, that when you do portion-control, force yourself to eat less, mask your appetite with tea, coffee, chewing gum, soups and fibre gels, success, even on the path of weight loss, becomes elusive.

And so we have the Mental Meal Map to our rescue, a simple tool that anyone can use to understand their appetite and learn how much to eat.

It has four steps:
- Step 1 – Visualize how much would you like to eat
- Step 2 – Serve yourself half of that amount
- Step 3 – Take double the time to eat the meal
- Step 4 – If still hungry, start again from Step 1

Start using the Mental Meal Map for at least one main meal every day. The Mental Meal Map is also extremely useful when you are eating out in restaurants or at weddings and party buffets.

> ## HOW MUCH TO EAT?
> ### Portions and Proportions
>
> **Portions**
> - Appetite varies due to many factors
> - Can't fix a portion size as standard
>
> Instead, use the **Mental Meal Map**
>
> 1. Visualise how much you want to eat
> 2. Serve yourself half of that amount
> 3. Eat slowly and take double the time
> 4. If still hungry, start from Step 1
>
> **Proportions**
> - All time-tested meals have roughly a 3:2:1 proportion of grains: dal/sabzi: pickle/salad/curd
> - This allows for optimum digestion and assimilation of nutrients
>
> Use the **Meal Proportion Map** for your meals
>
> - 15% Pickle, Papad, Salad, Curd, etc.
> - 35% Dal, Meat, Sabzi
> - 50% Rice, Roti, Bhakri, Millets

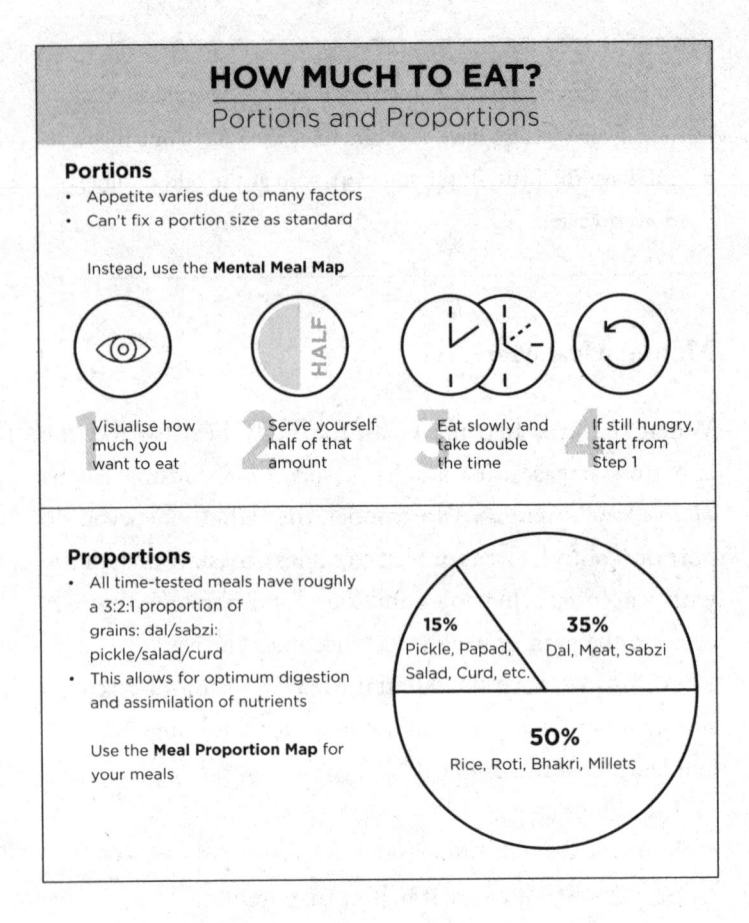

There is a time-tested formula for 'how to eat' also – the cornerstones of which are 'sit, silence, senses, slow'. I recommend you practice this 4S formula too. Start with once a week, build it to once a day, and soon enough, in all your meals you will stop eating before you get full.

Bhimsen Joshi, the greatest Indian classical singer ever, was also known for his love for cars and driving. Once he was on the road with Sudhir Gadgil, a well-known compere. The side-view mirror of the Mercedes that Panditji was driving almost brushed against a truck. Gadgil ducked out of fear for his life. '*Ghabru naka Gadgil, chukun sadi la haath lagel pan maandi touch honar nahi.*' (Don't worry Gadgil, I may brush against a saree in my oversight but will never go as off-track as touching the thigh.) That's the power of the daily *riyaaz*, lesser errors whether with food or sur.

See what you eat vs showing what you eat

On my Instagram, I often post pics of my food plate. First thing people notice is that it is silver.

'How does she eat so little?' Is the other thing they say. What you see is all there is (WYSIATI) is a common bias of the mind.[9] (Read *Thinking, Fast and Slow* by Daniel Kahneman.) Only with age and experience does one learn that there is more to see than what is being shown (be it a house hunt, job hunt or simply a first date). Displays are often a distraction from the real deal – we know that, but we forget it when we are on social media. When I click pictures of my thali, I place my food in a manner that looks attractive. It depicts the proportions in which I eat but not necessarily the portions. I plate my food in a manner that there is space between every item, so that every preparation is seen clearly. And after I am done posting, I will help myself to second helpings. I have explained this often, but maybe it's time to carry this disclaimer: 'Pic for representation purposes only. Doesn't depict the actual meal size of the said individual. You are encouraged to eat as per your appetite, and while you are at it may we also ask you to put your phone aside?'

6

What's not *ghar ka khaana*

UPF – the *anti-ghar ka khaana*

What is that one food whose consumption is growing fastest in the world amongst Indian youth? What is that one food which is directly linked to every single non-communicable disease, from diabetes to blood pressure to cancer and mental health? Actually, it is a trick question because the food in question – UPF (ultra-processed foods) – is not even real food.[10]

When Brazilian food scientist Carlos Monteiro and his team were researching the cause behind the obesity epidemic in Brazil, they came across a strange fact – households with more amount of salt, butter, sugar, in their kitchens, were in general healthier than others. This flew in the face of the conventional wisdom of that time – that the culprits were some problem nutrients in the food we consumed. What gives?

The presence of salt, sugar and butter was an indicator that those households were cooking more at home and eating less packaged and processed foods. This was one of the many facts that eventually led the team to come out with the NOVA classification of foods, where for the first time nutrition science clearly stated that it is the processing that is the problem, not the individual nutrients.

The NOVA classification

It is a framework that divides all the foods we eat into four categories based on the amount of processing they undergo.

Group I, includes 'unprocessed or minimally processed foods', like whole fruits and vegetables, grains, millets, beans and legumes, nuts, milk, eggs and cuts of meat.

Group II, or 'processed culinary ingredients', include cooking oils, butter, lard, sugar and salt.

Group III, or 'minimally processed foods', are often made by combining group I and group II ingredients into things like homemade breads, desserts, sautés, canned fish, bottled veggies and other dishes.

Group IV, or 'ultra-processed foods', are defined as formulations of ingredients that result from a series of industrial processes, including dyes, flavours, emulsifiers, certain sugars like fructose and other ingredients *rarely or never found in home kitchens*. This includes foods such as breakfast cereals, soft drinks, energy drinks, juices, and packaged snacks like chips, biscuits, cookies, reconstituted meat products, instant noodles, breads, frozen or long-shelf-life meals, etc.

Technical classification aside, here is my practical classification of food into four categories:

- **Group 1 – Home food:** food cooked in your kitchen, using a medley of ingredients that are a combination of fresh and perishable (veggies, milk products, etc.,) and non-perishables (millets, grains, legumes, pulses, spices, seeds, etc.). Ingredients that come together when cooked to reflect family and regional heritage and individuality. Food that calls your name, food that you return home to; food that is simple and uplifting.

    As we discussed earlier, home food should be 80 per cent of all the food that you eat. For the remaining 20 per cent, check below.

- **Group 2 – Gourmet food:** Food that you eat in posh restaurants/cool cafes or call for at home or have a chef cater for you. Food that you have developed a taste and liking for but isn't from your region or even the continent. But this food, too, is honest to the time-tested rules of the cuisine it belongs to.

- **Group 3 – Fun food:** Food that is world-famous in your region, not available anywhere else, has a local name. It's the street food of your region (and sometimes you make it at home, too). It makes you feel good when you eat it, has no ads but all the rich and famous of your area eat there/eat it. It isn't expensive but is not cheap either and, with time, the price may have gone up.

- **Group 4 – Junk food**: Food that is available globally, but now adapted to local taste buds, using masala formula, etc. Has ads, jingles, celeb endorsements, aggressive marketing and pricing to maximize reach. It is cheap and, with time, the price stays the same, but the size of the pack may have reduced (shrinkflation). Profit at the bottom of the pyramid.

The 20 per cent non-ghar ka khaana should mostly be from the fun and gourmet food categories, keeping the junk food to the bare minimum if you can't entirely avoid it.

Mother's love

My client was a young Kutchi boy working in the Bay Area – big money, pretty wife but *saala IBS se jeena haraam*. Slowly and steadily, we had worked at it, and now he had predictable motions, better digestion and reduced pain. Then the Covid lockdown lifted and his parents travelled to meet him. His mother carried with her his favourite bakarwadi. I planned for him to eat one every evening at chai time with his parents.

'I don't understand how you allow this,' said his wife to me. Some rich wives scold the consultants instead of their husbands. '*Aap toh videos mein kehte ho, jitna packet khulta hai, utna pet fulta hai.* Our basement is full of junk food but I was not saying anything to him. *Khane do jitna khana hai*, once the program starts, he has to stop.'

What's not *ghar ka khaana*

'See Mamta, he's not eating that junk food at all. But what his mother has brought is not just bhakarwadi. *Yeh pyaar, mohobbat aur ashirwaad hai.* Our parents are not with us forever, *ek time aisa bhi ayega ke apna favourite khaana laane wala ya even jaan ne wala koi nahi rahega.* Now he's eating just one a day, at a specific time, sipping chai with Mummy. It will be such a feel-good factor even for her that he's able to eat his favourite food and not make a run to the loo. It will boost her confidence about her son's health, it will teach him that one is good, two is too much. And one week *ke baad*, he won't even feel like eating it, so don't stress.'

The thing is that people often wonder how much is too much. The answer to that question is that **everything that is mindless is too much**, even if it's just one bite or scoop. So even when it comes to 'packaged food', if it's the specialty of your region, if you are sharing it with your own people, if its evoking nostalgia, love, laughter and tears, by all means go ahead and indulge.

But if it's packaged food that's available globally, that someone put in your room or flight seat as a freebie, that you are mindlessly chomping on because you are bored or watching TV, stop yourself. It's a no-brainer, really.

Food politics

We often use food to send a message – all the time, really. When we deprive ourselves of the foods we love, we tell ourselves that we are not worthy enough. When we allow ourselves the food we eat, even an extra helping, we tell ourselves that we are open to love and that we trust ourselves.

When we stop someone from accessing food that a loved one has sent/prepared, even if it's for 'health' reasons, we are simply being passive-aggressive. And we are being silly, petty too. But by allowing our partners to eat what their friends and families have got for them, we allow them the ability to receive love from all the ones who matter. We cannot possibly be everything to one person – parent, partner, child, bff, etc. It may be a romantic idea, but it is exhausting. It puts too much pressure on us and on the relationship.

My relationship advice to the young people I work with is just this – *khaane and khilaanewala ladka/ladki/family dhoondo. Baaki paisa, naam, hum khud kama sakte hain magar pyar se khilaanewale log important asset class hain.*

For a list of junk foods and their health-washed versions, see table on page 219.

Section 3

Commonsense Eating and Living

Ghar ka khaana

a.k.a

Home-cooked food

a.k.a

Dietary pattern

a.k.a

Local, seasonal, traditional

a.k.a

The commonsense diet

7

The food plan you can depend on

Ergonomics was one of my favourite subjects at college. Sports science and nutrition was then a newly launched course. Mine was the first batch, textbooks were non-existent, and we were dependent on external faculty to teach a whole lot of subjects – exercise physiology, ergonomics, sport psychology, etc. For ergonomics, we would go to the Industrial Development Centre at IIT-Bombay.

The whole point of ergonomics is to improve efficiency while reducing energy expenditure. This was late nineties, and I have literally watched experiments at the centre where doing *jhadu–katka* (mopping) changed from a sitting to a standing position. It allowed for more area to be covered, cleaned almost as well as the more classical squat down and reduced energy expenditure for the worker. A less tired worker is always a good thing. If the activity is not exhausting, compliance is better and efficiency is improved. So, how heavy a bat needs to be for hitting a sixer, how tall a chair should be for women workers, etc., is all ergonomics.

But why I am telling you this is because Mumbai has this project called the skywalk, which is for pedestrians to walk on. These are elevated walkways, mostly right outside railway stations, where you can walk freely without the danger of being hit by a car or bike almost all the way to the main road/highway. And yet you will find the skywalks empty and the public walking below, dodging cars, bikes, crossing busy roads and risking their lives.

If you don't know ergonomics, you are likely to think they lack the will and discipline to get home safely. But when you know better, you know that this is the outcome of poor design.

Firstly, people don't just walk home. They shop on their way, especially women. From daily vegetables, groceries, etc., all the chores are done between office and home. And all the shops are by the road. Secondly, there are no escalators to the skywalks, so you are not just making the daily walk back less efficient but also more tiring. And thirdly, if the skywalks are almost empty, it's dangerous because this is exactly where the molester will stand in wait for you.

You get design wrong when you don't account for the main thing. The main thing is that roads are built to move people, not just cars and bikes. Similarly, **the main thing a diet should do is to improve health; weight loss is secondary**. It's the car on the road. It can wait for its turn but allow the pedestrian to safely cross first. A diet that puts weight loss first will always cost you in terms of health. Like the skywalk, it will be an eye sore that didn't serve the purpose it was meant for.

> **Handa Sir**
>
> Prof. Sunil Handa, who taught one of the most coveted courses on entrepreneurship at IIM-A, says that he always blesses his students with a small health problem when they are about to graduate. Nothing serious, but enough that it gets them to realign their priorities and bring their focus to what is important – their health. The valuation of the many businesses that he has mentored and nurtured is worth over ₹10 lakh crore. 'Even hearing this makes me feel so happy, Sir. Doing this must have brought you so much happiness, I can't even imagine. And I also cannot imagine the number of people who will turn up for your funeral when you die.' I was saying this to him when we were taking a break from climbing a particularly steep slope on the Bara Banghal trek. 'Ha, ha, ha,' he laughed. 'You, Rujuta, are not just my dietitian or like my daughter, you are my dadi.' Best compliment I have ever received.

Diet design

A design fit is the most important predictor of compliance and therefore of success. So, if long flights, meetings, late hours, whatever else, are an occupational hazard, you need a diet plan that accounts for it all. That lets the body take it all on and thrive, and still be in a mode to sleep tight at night and get a twenty–thirty minutes workout squeezed in the morning. Life is not about looking like John Abraham, it's about looking like yourself. Because when we lose health, we actually do begin to look unlike ourselves.

So, how do you define a good diet design? One that you would use over and over again without getting tired of it. One that you want your children to adopt too. Because it is cost effective and improves the efficiency of your day-to-day life. It also accommodates for the holiday, the unexpected guests, the shaadi, or even tragedies. A successful diet, as we saw in the previous section, is something that you stay on till the end of time. Sustainability is at the core of its design.

And so, like every design, it must recognize the user and the problem, and then offer a suitable solution. Most importantly, the solution must not require the user to go out of her way to access it. Only then is it useful.

A food plan you can depend on

The Indian thought believes that all that is in the *pind* (individual or inside) is in the *brahmanda* (world or, outside). If the *pancha tatvas* that make the world are space, air, fire, water and earth, then they are represented in the body as *vata* (space and air), *pitta* (fire and water) and *kapha* (earth). And it is food that aligns the body and keeps the inside and outside in sync. Or it is food that is the link between the pind and the brahmanda. Food is called *anna* in Sanskrit, the English translation of which is something you consume but can consume you in return.

The confusion, conflict with food is a representation of being consumed by food. Consuming food is an act of human pleasure, uncomplicated and complete. Here's a guide to re-introducing the pleasures of eating wholesome meals back into our lives.

Feel free to modify it based on your region, heritage and tastes. This plan is kid-friendly.

On Waking Up	Breakfast
– a banana or any fresh fruit – handful of soaked nuts and dry fruits – Overnight soaked raisins with 1–2 kesar strands (PMS)* *A healthy start sets the tone for the day.* ** From our Ease PMS study*	– Poha, upma, idli, dosa, paratha, egg and pav, etc. – Deep-fried vada, poori or kachori (once a week) *Homemade nashta helps keep your blood sugars and moods steady through the day.*
Mid-Morning	**Lunch**
– Nimbu, kokum or amla sherbet. – Can also have coconut water or chaas here – Fresh fruit – A handful of nuts *Lack of hydration leads to sugar cravings post lunch. Replace one chai or coffee at work with a hydrating drink or a fresh fruit.*	– Roti or rice + sabzi (or meat) + dal and ghee. Finish with a glass of chaas. – Can add* – achaar, chutney, dahi, salad or kachumber Keep main things to 3 or even 2. ** Not counted in the 2-3 main items.*

Evening Snack*	Dinner
– Dry snacks like mathri, shankarpara, kurmura, chivda, chakli, khakra – Peanuts or chana or nuts – Seasonal specials like roasted shakarkandi or white corn – A sandwich, or roti-ghee-jaggery or a portion of your lunch – Chaat, once a week *A wholesome meal here helps you feel at ease and reduces chances of overeating at dinner.* * *Plan for this meal a week in advance.*	– khichdi or dal–rice, – roti–sabzi or bhakri-bhaaji (millets with sabzi) – phodni/tadka/vagharelo rice with an egg or paneer OR similar to lunch *Easy to cook and digest, and light on the stomach.*
At Bedtime	**5 good food habits**
– A cup of haldi milk* – Rice pej or rice kanji if you don't like milk *If you eat dinner early but get hungry later* *Can add – – Nutmeg, if you have weak digestion. – Gulkand in summer – Cashews for good sleep	1. Don't start your day with tea/coffee. 2. Avoid long gaps between meals. 3. Stop eating just before you become full. (Practice – sit, silence, slow, senses.) 4. Have ghee, fresh fruit and homemade chutney/pickle daily. 5. Finish your dinner 3 hours before bedtime. (Bring bedtime early, don't push dinner late.)

This is a framework that keeps you humane and in shape.

Regular *ghar ka khaana* – A practical guide

From what we have learnt about food combinations, proportions and portions and using the framework of the 'Food plan', here is an easy guide for regular *ghar ka khaana*.

Food	Options/ variations	How to eat	When and how often to eat
Rice (single polished or hand pounded or red rice)	Rice, poha, kurmura	Steamed rice, khichdi, pulao, biryani, poha, idli, dosa, ghavan, bhakri, papad, kurmura roasted like chivda or moori	1–3 times a day. As main meals or even snack. Celeb versions like biryani or pulao, once a week
Whole wheat	Flour from the chakki, rava, daliya	Chapati, parantha, upma, daliya, thepla, halwa, khakra	1–3 times a day. As main meals or even snack. Celeb versions – halwa or poori – once a week
Millets	Whole, or flour	Roti or bhakri, khichdi, thalipeeth, dosa, poori, kheer or raab, laddoo, papad, chikki	1–3 times a day. As part of main meals or as snacks. Celeb versions – kheer, halwa or poori – once a week

Food	Options/variations	How to eat	When and how often to eat
Pulses and dals	Whole, or atta	Dry chutney, laddoo, papad, dals, curries, chillas, dosa, wadi, pithla	1–3 times a day. As main meals or even snack Celeb versions like bhajji or dal pakwan – once a month
Legumes	Soaked and sprouted	Usal and curries, raitas, dry sabzi, dosa, kalan	1–3 times a day. As part of main meals or even snack
Vegetables	All kinds, including the hyper-local and wild varieties	Sabzi and curries, pickle, koshimbir (or kachumber)	1–3 times a day as part of main meals *Avoid on their own, in the version of salad bowls and smoothies
Yams and tubers	The wide varieties of suran, arbi, ratalu, tapioca, konfal, karande	Sabzi, curry, khichdi, kees, wada, roasted, kaap – shallow fry on tava	1–3 times a week. Part of main meal or snack Celeb versions like vada – once a month and undhiyo in season

Food	Options/variations	How to eat	When and how often to eat
Fruits	The local and seasonal ones, including the wild varieties	Fresh fruit, sherbet, milkshake, sweet preparations. Some like melon turned into a sabzi	1–3 times a day on their own. Best not to mix fruits. But you can have a banana with your meal. Celeb versions – aam ras in the mango season – daily or once a week. In-season fresh fruit like strawberry or sitaphal in milkshakes – daily or once a week
Nuts	Desi badam, walnut, pista, cashew	Eat them raw or as a garnish in sweet dishes or biryani/pulao, powdered and added to milk	1–2 times a day Also include a handful of peanuts or chana as a snack
Seeds	Flaxseed, methi seeds, aliv seeds, til, etc.	Chutney, tadka, laddoo, chikki, mukhwaas	1–2 times a day for chikki, laddoo; chutney versions and tadka will be more often than that Avoid the 'on its own' versions like seed shots

Food	Options/variations	How to eat	When and how often to eat
Spices	Ginger, garlic, haldi, soonth, jeera, ajwain, pepper, hing, cinnamon, etc.	Tadka, chutney, achaar, garnish, etc.	Daily – spices are small part of all Indian wholesome meals But avoid the 'on its own' versions like garlic pods or haldi shots
Dry fruit	Raisins, anjeer, dates, dry dates, jardalu or apricot	Eat them raw or as a garnish in sweet dishes or biryani/pulao, or add to milk	1–2 times a day Sweet dishes once a week
Fats and oils	Groundnut, til, mustard, coconut (kacchi ghaani or cold-pressed or filtered)	For tadka, for deep and shallow frying, garnishing dry chutneys and in preparations like kichu	Daily use as necessary in cooking. And enjoy the fresh garnishes and chutneys, 1–2 times a day.
Dairy products	Milk, dahi, chaas, ghee, butter, paneer	Can be had by themselves or as an accompaniment. Also a part of tadka, garnish, raitas, kadhi	Can be had on their own – milk to start and end the day Dahi and chaas as mid meals or as accompaniments to main meals, ghee or makhan as required with main meals

Food	Options/ variations	How to eat	When and how often to eat
			No problem if you would rather avoid dairy products, too.
Meat, fish, eggs		Curry, kebab, tava fry, part of biryani, pickles	As part of main meals but not on their own, except may be eggs
			(Range varies from 3 times a day to 3 times a week, as per your culture)
			No problem if you would rather avoid them.
Sugar	Sugarcane, jaggery, laal shakkar, white sugar, kakvi	To bring mithas to all things	Can add to tea/coffee/sherbets, as garnish on some sabzis or dals, and in homemade mithai
			Restrict to 3–6 tsp per day. Don't replace sugar with sweeteners

Please note that this list is not exhaustive but indicative. And many foods can be in more than one category, e.g. – peas are both a vegetable and a pulse. Til could be a seed or a source of fat. Have also added peanuts and chana, technically legumes, to nuts, for practical purposes. So, this is more like a practical checklist of sorts.

Zone of control

My client has a successful business across the seven seas; there's nothing that he cannot do. And yet, when his eighty-year-old mom came to visit him in Singapore and got sick, there was nothing he could do except cool his heels in the hospital waiting room. 'I would trade everything for her to be ok,' he said to me on the phone. 'She's going to be fine Dinesh, you hang in there.'

A few procedures and a close call later, she was fine and all set for discharge. She's been a client of mine too. A robust woman who plays cards from 3 p.m. to 8 p.m. and has different groups – rummy, bridge, etc. 'Body will slow down but *dimaag daudna chahiye*,' she had said to me. Planning her diet was fun because all her friends would host each other by turn from Monday to Friday, and there was the speciality of every house served with the evening chai – muthiya, dhokla, poha, etc.

Upon her discharge, the first question she asked her doctor was '*Ghar kab jaa sakti hu* and can I eat one mithai every day?' The doctor said, 'You are so fit, you can take the evening flight itself to Mumbai and not one but two mithai every day.' She looked at Dinesh and said to the doctor, 'Please tell him.' The doctor addressed Dinesh, 'You heard me, right?' Dinesh nodded.

His mother out of his sight was the last thing he wanted. 'I have a lot to do in Mumbai,' Dinesh's mom had argued with him. 'What do you have to do?' Pay salaries to her staff of seven and make monthly contributions to the five groups she played in. 'You can do that online,' Dinesh argued back.

'No, I can't,' said the mother. 'There's a lot that I do other than just pay money. But you think no one has any work other than you.' Then there's a driver's mom whom she had to take to her physician to check on her kidney stone, go with her friend to buy a necklace, and she had also committed to making muthiya for a relative's son. 'You will forget about me in two days and get busy with work, but people depend on me there.'

When people have a close call with death, there are only two things they wish for – shelter, to be back in the place they call home, and food, familiar and friendly/delicious food. These are two things that make us feel alive. And irrespective of how rich or poor we are, this is all we need. Also, we need to feel like we are needed, like we will be missed, and that tasks will be interrupted due to our absence. **Our comfort zone is our zone of control, where we are in charge of our home, food, and therefore life.**

8

Tracking progress

When science is allowed to function like it is meant to – to help us make informed decisions and overcome our intrinsic biases – it works exactly like common sense. You could say that even about business acumen or war strategy or personal relationships, *common sense must be our guide.* We must know what to ignore and what to focus our energy on. Common sense is like magic because the truth is often hidden in plain sight and the focus is on the distraction.

It's a bit like solving crimes. A good detective looks for patterns and uses that to anticipate and hopefully prevent the next crime. A serial dieter has a pattern too – of eliminating all that they enjoy eating. Every time, there's murder of taste and texture in the hope of a new cure or weight loss. Once you identify this pattern, you can stop yourself from going on the next diet and killing time and muscle.

'All right, I agree to everything, but can I actually lose weight if I continue to eat normally?' The answer is yes, hell yes. But slowly, steadily and sustainably. *Sustainable weight loss is 5–10 per cent of current weight per year.* If you commit to that, you can get there while living the full life you have planned for yourself. You can focus at work, have fun with family, the friendship of a community and a lot more, as you evolve into the real you. The one who realizes that the body is a vehicle with which to pursue and achieve all that one desires. And so, only losing weight is not going to be enough. I must also knock off inches on my waist, build more strength in my legs, be able to run for twenty minutes at a stretch, squat with at least my body weight and hold the Shirsasana for three minutes. The wish list is endless, and health is a moving goal post.

Tracking progress

So, I am going to let you in on my trade secret. *When I work with clients, I don't weigh them.* I don't own a weighing scale. It is lazy to weigh clients. Instead, we put them through a full fitness assessment. You can download home fitness tests from anywhere on the internet. They are standardized and easy to self-administer. These tests also act as a very good indicator of your overall metabolic health – i.e., hormonal health, heart health, blood sugar regulation, etc. – and give a much better idea of your fitness than the number on the weighing scale.

You need to check the following:
- Resting heart rate (RHR) – ideally, first thing on rising
- Strength – typically, number of squats per minute

- Stamina – step test for 3 mins
- Stability – how long can you hold the plank pose
- Flexibility – sit and reach for your toes
- Waist – circumference at the narrowest part
- Hips – circumference at the broadest part (for the waist-to-hip ratio)

This is easy because you will get a number for each. It is tangible, and all that you do is *keep your eyes on the progress you make, not on the actual numbers*. So, let's say you started the sit-and-reach test with being 8 inches away from your toes. Three months later, if your fingers are only 6 inches away from the toes, it is good progress.

Good is not 'Oh, now I can reach my toes.' It is, 'I am getting there.' Because once you do reach your toes, you are going to want to reach beyond them. That's a natural human tendency, as natural as wanting to go from 1bhk to 3bhk. But in our zest for it, if we forget to celebrate that we have a roof over our heads, then it's a long-term problem that a 3bhk won't solve, nor will a 5bhk with a rooftop swimming pool. We must learn to have basic gratitude.

It is the same with the waist-to-hip ratio. For men, the waist should be under 40 inches, and for women, under 36 inches. And then, for men, when you divide waist to hip, the ratio should be 0.8 to 1 and for women between 0.7 and 0.85. But let's say you are a woman who started with a waist of 43. Even if you got to 41 in three months it is good; 36 may be a long way to go and 28 is where you would like to be at, but if you don't celebrate the journey, 28 is not going to be a happy destination either.

The reason why 'I charge so much' is because we deliver more than just weight loss. People improve on their health and fitness first and the weight loss follows. This is the only way sustainability works. And no, it doesn't work the other way around. When you lose weight quickly, and when that is the primary focus, you also lose in terms of the number of squats you can do per minute, or your technique gets poorer as the strength from your legs is the first to go.

And the hips shrink but the waist stays or even increases, disturbing your waist-to-hip ratio, now actually putting you at a risk of developing metabolic diseases in the long run, even though you have lost weight. Your hamstrings get stiffer, so you may still reach your toes but the journey gets tougher. The core gets weaker over time, joints hurt, sleep goes, appetite fluctuates, moods swing. Not worth it at all.

Google and the role of healthy skepticism

Dr Sai Satish of Apollo Chennai, tells his team to not mock people for going on Google. 'They are sick and scared. If they are not irritating you, then you are doing something wrong. And if we are such a good team, we must be able to defend our line of treatment and explain it in a manner that is understood by the patient.' 'Skepticism must be encouraged', he says. 'You make less errors that way.'

> He also encourages the people he treats to seek a second opinion. Clarity only comes out of confusion.
>
> And my two cents here are: don't check your cardio's prescription with your dermat and vice versa. Get an expert in the same field to weigh in.

More data points

So, when you have to decide how good the diet plan you are on is, you must build more than one data point. Not just weight but strength, stamina, flexibility, stability, RHR, waist-to-hip ratio, etc. Measure them, track them – once every three months.

Along with that we should also track things we can't really count but can give a rating to – sleep, acidity, bloating and constipation, exercise compliance, period regularity, aches and pains, mood swings and sugar cravings. And thirdly, if you have any metabolic condition, track that too with blood tests, as prescribed by your doctor. So track your HbA1c, liver enzymes, lipid profile, TSH – whatever may be relevant in your case. And then take a wholesome view on how you are treating your body.

One of the things that I always tell my clients (one more trade secret) is that **your approach towards health and wealth should be mirror images of each other**. When it comes to wealth generation, work, etc., go hard at yourself. Push all boundaries, stay up all night, slog all day, think of nothing but the task at hand and go all mad about it.

But when it comes to health generation, weight loss and fitness, go easy. Respect the body and its limitations, get good sleep, skip the workout today if you haven't recovered from yesterday's, don't think about calories, weight, steps, all day. Stay sane. It's the only way to stay sensible and sustainable.

This I have to tell my clients because most of them are super achievers who wonder *ke agar duniya pe kaabu kar liya toh shareer pe kyu nahi*. They are almost embarrassed that they have had to sign up because how difficult can weight loss be? It is not, but you are on the wrong track. If you push too hard, your body will snap. And you don't want that. Remember the definition of health at the start of the book? The state where you forget about your body. The mother, the nap, the train, no flies on the face and, most importantly, safety of the baby. If we can get meditative with our bodies, then really, why not?

Ayu – vayu – payu

One of my clients, Ajay Lakahanpal, gifted me a copy of the principal Upanishads. The book gives the English translation of the Sanskrit text, word by word and then the full verse. I read two shlokas daily, that's my morning ritual. It doesn't have anyone's version of what the shlokas mean, it is simply telling us what the OG authors wrote. I love it. Every time it's like discovering a new reality. One of the shlokas has

> this equation – the more often you use your *payu* or feet, the stronger your *saman vayu* or digestive powers, and the longer your *ayu* or length of life. So the idea of daily steps is quite ancient, but unlike in the modern world, it's not prescriptive – 10k a day or whatever. It's a lot more commonsensical.
>
> Staying active makes you feel alive, improves your digestion and helps you feel light on your feet. You need to be on a food plan which, by default, helps you get more active and makes you feel like walking instead of taking a rick. Where you spring up on your feet to answer the doorbell instead of calling out to your house help.

So, even with tracking progress, don't track every single thing every single month. But list out about three outcomes max that you would want to stay on track with. So, if cravings are an issue, list the number of times you ordered food last-minute. If poor sleep is an issue, list the number of times you wake up in the night. If your stomach is an issue, list the number of times you needed a fibre supplement. And then, along with that, measure your waist and hip.

Do this every month and self-administer the fitness tests, or at least two of them, every three months. That way, whatever your goal is – whether it's improving your HbA1c, body weight, triglycerides, uric acid – it will be met in a sustainable manner. And how often should you weigh yourself? Once every three months. That much is more than enough to check on trends. Vigilance and not anxiety.

Guide to tracking progress

	Data points	How to track	How often
1. Things that can be measured	Resting heart rate Waist-to-hip ratio Weight Strength Stamina Flexibility Stability	Standard fitness tests, Tape measurements, etc.	Once in 3 months
2. Things that can be tracked but not measured	Sleep quality Acidity, bloating and constipation Sugar cravings Mood swings Exercise compliance Aches and pains Period regularity	Keep notes	Monthly
3. Metabolic conditions	HbA1c TSH BP Liver enzymes Lipid profile etc.	Lab tests	Only when relevant and as prescribed by your doctor

It's important to remember that all the health outcomes associated with weight loss will come your way only with improved body composition. Without improved waist-to-hip ratio, strength in the lower limbs, stability in the core, flexibility in the posterior chain, the risk of non-communicable diseases (NCDs), or for that matter even response to infectious diseases, will not change.

And when these improve, the risk drops significantly, even if body weight hasn't dropped yet. Health is a journey, not a destination. Focus on the trend, not the arrival. This is also the reason why train journeys are always more powerful and romantic than air travel. They allow you to enjoy the progress, take in the taste and fragrance of Vapi, Ratlam and Panipat before arriving at Amritsar.

Pharmaceutical or nutraceutical?

I went to vote on 23 November for the Maharashtra assembly elections. As I entered the polling area, I noticed one of the polling officers pouring tons of capsules from a fish oil bottle.

'*Kaay Sir,*' I asked, '*divsachya kiti?*' How many per day?
'Ten', he replied, 'twice a day.'

'Diabetes,' both of us said together and nodded, and I went ahead to show my Aadhaar card and cast my vote.

Does the pharma lobby exist? Yes. Are they here to make a profit? Yes. But they have a product that works. Administered the right way, with due diligence and care towards eating right, exercising and making lifestyle changes, you could potentially keep many problems away. Taking a pill and taking care of one's lifestyle are not mutually exclusive. They are both interventions for a good and healthy life.

So, stick it out with the basics. And track your parameters – what's happening to the waist-to-hip ratio, digestion, moods, etc. – and you will notice that your body is now regulating HbA1c better. Over time, you will notice that you need a smaller dose to stay within a good range, and are hopefully able to come off the drug too. If not, your worst case is that you are at the same dose for the next ten or fifteen years, enabled by your diverse diet and consistent exercise. And your heart, kidney, nerves, eyes, etc., are in a good shape too because of the healthy routine you have built.

Not taking the diabetes pill but taking a ton of nutraceuticals, twenty to thirty pills, is not going to keep pharma profits down. They make the supplements too and you are just keeping another vertical of theirs cash-rich.

9

Diet recalls and modifications

Getting to know you

'Ma'am, I am a diabetic', or 'I am 5'4" and 86 kgs' – that's not an introduction according to me. It tells me nothing about you. And, more importantly, it tells me nothing about what I should do with your diet. What should I change? What should remain the same? What needs to be brought back? What needs to be removed?

When people sign up with me, I always ask them to write their expected program outcomes. Their top three, in no order of priority. My work involves designing or planning a diet to meet those outcomes and set timelines for the same. We call it the 'Getting to Know You' sheet. People hate writing it because it also means documenting their health history, telling us when they were at their fittest, how the lockdown affected them, how their sleep and exercise are, etc.

Surprisingly, almost no one writes that they want to lose weight as one of their top three expected outcomes. It is amazing that once people have had the time to think and reflect on why they are making an investment of time and resources into getting healthier, they want different things from losing weight. They want to feel more energetic, sleep better, prepare better for ageing, climb Patalsu or Kilimanjaro without being overtly tired, and more.

The fact is that we are all here for a limited time. When we understand this, we rationalize the amount of time and bandwidth we are willing to spend on chasing numbers. A sustainable diet is the one that allows us to take our focus off the weight chart and blood report but never let them forget that we are watching, just like the mother with her kid at Haridwar station.

Case studies

Here are a few real-life diet recalls. Typically, we ask our clients to write down the details of their entire day in real time and send us this recall for three days. We have shortlisted diverse profiles; descriptions have been changed out of respect for privacy, everything else has been told exactly like it happened (my ode to "Fargo"). If you think it is looking exactly like your recall, that's because so many of us make the exact same mistakes with food. Alongside them are our recommendations to show how even very small modifications to one's diet, exercise and lifestyle can lead to steady and sustainable improvements.

In fact, my clients often wonder 'but mostly I was eating like this only earlier,' when they see improvements in their health. So, other than adding this here and removing that from there, I have done nothing much. Building a sustainable diet means not needing you to do a dance and drama every time you want to use it. Small changes that don't take away from your way of life are the most powerful because of the compounding effect they offer.

Compounding

A fund manager client of mine was once in her doctor's waiting room. She asked the compounder what she does for her investments. 'Nothing, there's nothing left at the end of the month,' she said. 'Are there ₹500 left at the end of every month?' '₹600,' replied the compounder. 'Ok, give it to me', said my client. ₹600 every month and three years later, she had built a portfolio of close to a lakh. 'How do I have so much money?' asked the compounder. *'Nanu nanu, motu thai che,'* my client replied. Small things turn big over time.

We are able to suggest these small changes only because we get to really know our clients over time. Thirty minutes one-on-one, week after week. Seeing them through their menstrual phases, launching IPOs, going through mergers, marriages and more, allows us a unique insight into the small things that will make the tide smoother. Honestly, people making quick recommendations as to what you must do or making big changes by just watching viral reels is silly and wasteful to say the least.

I am hoping that these examples will guide you with regard to the kind of small changes you can make in your own diet and lifestyle to enjoy huge gains in your health portfolio in the long run.

#1

Who: A vibrant Marwari homemaker in her fifties trying to navigate her menopause and falling prey to an array of misleading diet advice in the process. She has spent the last 30 years on diets and tried every latest weight loss aid (including Ozempic). As her BP began to fluctuate, palpitations and anxiety attacks became frequent and the list of pills piled up, we were, as I've heard many of our clients say, her last resort.

Ailments: Frequent stomach upsets and infections, hot flashes, a sudden increase in weight, depression for five years, knee pain, fluctuating BP

Goals: feel better, sleep better, not wake up sweating

Day 1	Day 2	Day 3
10.45 a.m. – Small elaichi banana	8.30 a.m. – Banana	9.30 a.m. – 1 sourdough toast and tea
11.30 a.m. – Plant protein (1 scoop) with chaas, papaya and mosambi, tea	9.30 a.m. – 1 sourdough bread toast and tea	12 p.m. – Plant protein (1 scoop) chaas, papaya (small bowl) and 1 mosambi
2.15 p.m. Lunch – apple cider in water, salad (1 bowl) with moong sprouts, arugula, red and green cabbage, and paneer grilled sandwich with capsicum, onion and cilantro, (2 slices of bread) + 1/4th cup of tea with just a teaspoon of milk and no sugar	12 p.m. – Plant protein (1 scoop) with chaas and fruits	2 p.m. – Salad (1 bowl), 2 laal masoor dal chilla with dahi
	2.30 p.m. – Salad, chawli, dahi and 1 sourdough toast	3 p.m. – Cold coffee with Splenda and a dash of oat milk
	4.30 p.m. – Cold coffee with Splenda and a dash of oat milk	5.45 p.m. – Tea and chana kurmura
5 p.m. – Cold coffee with Splenda and a dash of oat milk	6 p.m. – Karela, amla, haldi juice and 4 almonds, 1 walnut	9.30 p.m. – 1 big bowl of salad and vatana and kulcha
6.30 p.m. – Bitter gourd juice with amla and amba haldi, 4 almonds and 4 walnuts	8.45 p.m. Dinner – 1 big bowl of salad and 1 and half paratha with matar paneer	
8.30 p.m. Dinner – 1 carrot, 1 cucumber, missal with 1 pav		

Diet recalls and modifications

Observations: She tries to include every influencers' secret recipe to weight loss, from anti-inflammatory diets to green juices, and every new product that is on the market. There is fear of sugar, of carbs – of a full meal, basically. Some local, traditional food items are included too, but without the time-tested combinations, and only out of greed for their goodness. The desperate bids have led to a weak gut, poor sleep and a tougher transition to menopause.

Recommendations	
1	Add rice-based meals (dal rice/pulao/kadhi rice) at dinner 2 days a week to allow digestion to get better
2	Replace Splenda with regular white sugar in coffee, and oat milk with regular milk
3	Remove vegetable juices/methi pani/amla shots, etc. from 4–6 p.m. and, instead, have a wholesome meal
4	Avoid eating large quantities of salad; eat it as a small part of the main meal and don't use it to curb appetite
5	Regulate lunch time to 2 p.m. max, and dinners to 8 p.m. and keep them basic
Progress	In 6 months:
1	The waist size dropped 4 inches, the navel dropped 2 inches
2	Her moods got better, she was able to taper down the dose of her anti-depressant and her doctor was only happy to help
3	Her knee pain became a thing of the past and she began doing body weighted full squats during her exercise sessions
4	Intensity and frequency of night sweats dropped, allowing her unbroken sleep for 4–5 hours at a stretch

#2

Who: A young, driven doctor in his mid-thirties, practising in the US. Night shifts, day shifts were his routine life. An overachiever, he has been a hardworking boy since childhood and believes weight loss is about will power, discipline and behavioural shifts. He blamed his erratic schedule and felt that with time it was getting harder for him to drop the weight no matter how hard he pushed.

Ailments: Depression, anxiety, IBS

Goals: Reduce body fat, increase lean muscle mass, feel more energetic

Day 1	Day 2	Day 3
2:30 a.m. – 1 black coffee and 1 cup chole	1:00 a.m. – drank whey protein shake	2:00 a.m – had snack box: some grapes, peanuts, cheese
6:00 a.m. – 1 CLIFF bar, 1 protein bar (perfect bar)	1:30 a.m. – drank 1 cup of black coffee	9:00 a.m – 5 methi thepla, 1 cup desi yogurt and 1 cup palak paneer
Slept from 8 a.m.–3 p.m.	7:00 a.m. Left from work	9:30 a.m – sleep
4:00 p.m. – 1 vegetable burrito, chips, salsa, cheese stick, 1 Sabra hummus cup	7:30 a.m. – ate couple of chocolate cubes	1:30 p.m. – woke up
	8:00 a.m. – ran 10k	2:30 p.m. – 1.5 bajra rotla, 2 cup sev tameta nu shak
	11:00 a.m. – drank 1 cup of Indian tea, ate 2 cups of chori nu shak with one cup of yogurt, 1 pack Maggi	4:30 p.m. 1 cup Indian tea

1:00 a.m. – 1 cup chole, 1 protein bar (perfect bar) 2:00 a.m. – ½ bag Chex Mix 3:00 a.m. – 1 cup chole	Slept from 11:30 a.m. – 4 p.m., woke up 2–3 times for using restroom 4:15 p.m. – drank one cup of Indian tea 5:00 p.m. – went to work 11:00 p.m. – came back from work 11:30 p.m. – ate 2 cups of chori nu shak with one cup of yogurt, 1 packet of Chex Mex. 12:00 a.m. – napped	7:00 p.m. – black coffee 8:00 p.m. – 1 bottle whey protein 9:00 p.m. – a 45-minute treadmill run 9:50 p.m. – 10-minute strength training 10:20 p.m. – 2 cup baingan bharta, 1 bajra rotlo, 1 whey protein bottle 11:00 p.m. – went for night shift for work

Observations: Whether it was a day shift or a night shift, he ate no more than two wholesome meals in the entire day in order to keep his diet low-cal. The rest was a barrage of tea/coffee/ready-to-eat protein bars/protein shakes. And when it was an emotionally draining day, the cheetos/maggie/chex-mex would come out, making it a bad boy–good boy routine; days which were 'good' where he barely ate led to days which were very bad with binge eating episodes.

Recommendations	
1	Add grains like rice with chole/pita with hummus for more balanced meals and to avoid erratic hunger during the day
2	Remove all the packaged versions – protein shakes/bars/Maggi/Chex Mex/Cheetos, etc., from home pantry
3	Replace protein bars and stock up peanuts/chikki/yogurt/chana, etc., for in-between meals
4	Avoid more than 1 black coffee during the night shift and include a more hydrating drink like nimbu sherbet or buttermilk or a fresh fruit
5	Regulate the number of take-outs in a week to 2–3 times (50 % of his current number) and get food from a local aunty instead
Progress	In 3 months:
1	Lost 2 inches at his navel and dropped a size overall
2	Didn't feel as exhausted post his exercise, his compliance with his running got better and his calf pain had disappeared
3	Eventually, he rediscovered his love for food and even employed a cook to come twice a week so he could rely much less on packaged foods and have more access to *ghar ka khaana*.

#3

Who: An ambitious 27-year-old event planner who was worried sick that the tastings and entertaining – a routine part of her work – was going to make her fat and old very quickly. She was also harrowed by constantly having to coordinate with multiple agencies at her work.

Ailments: None. But there were mood swings, having just gone through a bad breakup.

Goals: Get rid of cravings, fat loss, better mood and mental health, especially while dealing with unrealistic expectations of clients

Day 1	Day 2	Day 3
Wake up 8 a.m.	Wake up 8 a.m.	Wake up 8 a.m.
8:15 a.m. – Black coffee	8:15 a.m. – Black coffee	8:15 a.m. – Black coffee
12 noon – Black coffee	Got to office by 10:30 and was there all day	Got to office by 10:30 a.m. and was there all day
1:30 p.m. Lunch – 2 Edamame truffle dumplings 1 Crystal dumpling 2 Chilean sea bass mooli roll – no carb 1 Prawn wrapped in spinach – no carb 2 pieces of crispy prawn cheung fun 2 spoons of egg fried rice 1 piece tenderloin 3–4 French beans	12 noon – Black coffee 1:30 p.m. – Leftover khao suey from previous night 3:30 p.m. – Handful of makahana	12 noon – Black coffee 1:00 p.m. – ½ Paneer bhurji roll with salad (lettuce and cucumber with mustard olive oil dressing)

4:00 p.m. – a few pieces of toast with caviar/cheese and bowl of boiled corn Went home after lunch and worked all evening 7:00 p.m. – 1 bowl bhaji (Pav bhaji) no bread 8:30 p.m. – 2 bowls of khao suey – Little noodles, chicken broth – lots of veggies – fried garlic and onions, ordered in from my fav restaurant. 3 glasses of red wine 10:30 p.m. – a bowl of pasta with cheese and chilli oil/pepper – I get increasingly hungry around this time and always crave rice, noodles or pasta Had chips, a glass of coke and some popcorn while watching a romcom Slept at 1 a.m.	7:30 p.m. – 1 paneer bhurji roll 9:30 p.m. – 2 bowls of daal, 1 pomfret fillet, 1 rice bhakri, 1 bowl of salad, 2 glasses of wine Got home Slept by 11.30 p.m.	4:20 p.m. – Lunch – ½ paneer bhurji roll with salad (lettuce and cucumber with mustard olive oil dressing) and two bites of dessert tasting 5:20 p.m. – a handful of makhana 6:15 p.m. – Went for a dessert tasting, five bites of dessert during tasting 7:15 p.m. – Came home, had one bowl of rice with prawn curry 8:30 p.m. – Had dinner – 1 almond flour pizza with sausages, cheese, onion, jalapeno, mushroom, peppers and 1 bowl of salad 2 glasses of red wine Ended up stalking my ex, sorry! Needed a bowl of ice-cream after. Slept by 1 a.m.

Observations: If you look closely, you see her keeping herself hungry for the first half of the day. As the day progresses, she tries to eat 'low carb' or 'no carb' and finally ends the day with pasta, pizza and wine, feeling guilty and disappointed (only to repeat the same cycle the next day). She is also keeping a 16-hour fasting window, so the first meal is often 3–4 hours after reaching office, making it difficult for her to not shout at everyone who crosses her path and needing two large coffees to make it till 2 p.m. Sometimes, she wonders if she has turned into a permanent bridezilla herself.

Recommendations	
1	Add a breakfast of parantha or eggs and toast before leaving home/on reaching office
2	Replace late night snacks with a haldi milk
3	Remove ice-cream, chips and other UPFs – limit them to 1 serving a week, max
4	Avoid having leftover dinner for the next day's breakfast and lunch, especially if it is from outside
5	Regulate the wine to maximum once a week and eat dinner before you drink
Progress	**In 3 months:**
1	Waist and navel measurements dropped by 2 inches each
2	Lower body strength improved from 13 squats to 20 squats in a minute, giving her butt a round and toned look. The plank went from 20 seconds to a full 50 seconds, almost pushing a minute

3	Cravings disappeared and so did the bloating
4	She stopped stalking her ex and began to enjoy her work a lot more

#4

Who: Delhi-based lawyer in his early sixties. Reluctantly gave into his daughter's wish for him to be on the program. With her wedding around the corner, she thought it was time she got her father the guidance he needed. She described him as a 'highly functioning alcoholic'.

Ailments: Pre-diabetic, BP, but not started on the drug yet

Goals: Stamina for daughter's wedding, client meetings abroad, Ladakh bike trip with the boys

Day 1	Day 2	Day 3
5.15 a.m. – woke up	5.30 a.m. – woke up	6 a.m. – woke up
5.20 a.m. – big mug of masala chai	5.40 a.m. – big mug of masala chai	6.30 a.m. – big mug of masala chai
5.30 a.m. – sat down to work at home office	5.45 a.m. – sat down to work at home office	6.45 a.m. – no workout as long day
6.45 a.m. – freshened up and got ready for workout	6.30 a.m. – freshened up and got ready for workout	8 a.m. – slice of brown bread with cheese
7.30–8.30 a.m. – PT at home, back exercises	7.30–8.20 a.m. – yoga at home	10 a.m. – got ready to go for recce for daughter's wedding venue
8.35 a.m. – salt lime water	8.20 – salt lime water	

Diet recalls and modifications

8.40 a.m. – got ready for work	8.25 a.m. – got ready for work	3 p.m. – chicken kebab, butter chicken, black dal, roti, falooda, at friend's restaurant
9.10 a.m. – left for work in my car (driver driven)	8.40 a.m. – left for work in my car (driver driven)	5.30 p.m. – left in the car (driver) for shopping
9.45 a.m. – in the office (standing desk, moving around as much as possible)	9.15 a.m. – in the office 10.40 a.m. – black coffee	7.30 p.m. – back home, freshening up
10.45 a.m. – black coffee	1 p.m. – quinoa salad bowl	8 p.m. – 3 small whiskey
1.30 p.m. – grilled fish with fresh salad and a diet coke	4.30 p.m. – 4 chicken nuggets with coke zero	9.30 p.m. – keto pizza
5 p.m. – 2 chicken nuggets with black coffee	7 p.m. – back home	10 p.m. – off to bed, asleep in about 15 minutes.
6.30 p.m. – 2 small whiskey, mixed nuts, entertaining clients	8.45 p.m. – 3 small whiskey (family get together at home)	12,424 steps per fitbit
8 p.m. – back home	9.45 p.m. – 3 slices of hand tossed pizza, little dal makhani and paneer matar	
9 p.m. – chilli chicken and palak mushroom, small bowl of gajar halwa	11.20 p.m. off to bed	
9.45 p.m. – retire to bed and fall asleep in some time (about 15 minutes)	7,806 steps per fitbit	
8,825 steps per fitbit		

Observation: In a bid to regulate his sugars and get more benefit from his workouts, he had replaced all his meals with protein. But without the addition of carbs, his body lost out on the 'protein sparing effect' and failed to build adequate strength and muscle. The drinking was frequent, both socially and at work during client meetings. He was also resistant to adding wholesome meals because of time constraints and diets that had 'worked like magic' in the past.

Recommendations	
1	Add a banana pre-workout
2	Replace salad and grilled fish lunch with roti, sabzi and dahi
3	Remove colas and have shikanji (nimbu sherbet), bael or amla sherbet
4	Avoid keto pizza and just eat regular pizza once a week – 2 slices
5	Regulate drinks to 2 a week and only with clients, not friends
Progress	**In 6 months:**
1	16 squats in a minute to 24 full range deep squats 21 incline pushups to 7 full pushups 1.19-minute plank to 2.05-minute plank hold
2	Stamina on bike rides went up and avoiding drinks on flights helped reduce jet lags and fatigue
3	He dropped 3 inches on his waist, 2 inches on his navel and the hip remained the same, making for a better waist to hip ratio.

#5

Who: 30-year-old software professional with long working hours who had recently moved outside the country. A year ago, she did an Ayurvedic diet to balance the hormones and get smooth, pain-free periods. But it wasn't a fit to her lifestyle and left her exhausted with debilitating cramps. The doctors scared her that she may have endometriosis, and her confidence dropped lower than ever.

Ailments: Painful cramps and heavy bleeding during periods

Goals: Smooth and pain-free periods – 'Only 1 goal I have. I cannot go on with this pain for 30 more years.'

Weekday	Weekend
7.30 a.m. – wake up and have moringa powder in water	7:30 a.m. – wake up and drink cinnamon and methi seed water
9 a.m. – tea with almond milk (regular milk is not allowed) and Marie biscuit	8:10 a.m. – 1 cup tea + 1 marie biscuit
11 a.m. – pomegranate with soaked chia seeds	9:10 a.m. – muskmelon shake in oat milk with chia seeds
2 p.m. – Barley water before the meal lauki with minimal masala, rice, moong dal	12:00 p.m. – bathed
	1:30 p.m. – went out for stroll along the beach
	1:45 p.m. – 1 apple
5 a.m. – Nimbu paani with ginger juice and turmeric paste with jaggery, elaichi powder and a pinch of salt added	2 p.m. – made lunch
	2:15 p.m. – half vanilla cupcake while cooking
6 p.m. – Methi pulao	2:30 p.m. – 2 katori sambhar, 1.5 katori rice, 3 tbsp rajma curry

9.30 p.m. – choco-strawberry vegan and sugar free ice cream Slept by 10 p.m.	3 p.m. – took out clothes from washing machine and hung them on the cloth stand 4–6:15 p.m. – nap on daybed 6:15 p.m. – 1 pc Kaju katli 7 p.m. – avocado toast 7:20 p.m. – made Nutella toast (craving for sweet) 7:25 p.m. – ate Nutella toast 8:00 p.m. – pending office work 8:30 p.m. – 2 whisky sour, vegan burger and french fries (craving salty and fried and tasty food) 11 p.m. – 1 chocolate espresso vegan and sugar free ice cream Slept at 1 a.m.

Observations: Her ayurvedic diet allowed only moong and no other pulses, not even tur, plus lauki in every meal, different shots during the day and limited fruit intake, only pomegranate. An integrative medicine person asked her to go vegan, shift to mock meat, drink smoothies and eat fresh salads instead of grains. The conflicting views had left her more confused than ever, so her recall had a bit of both, plus a few odd things she picked from social media. Her weekdays left her exhausted, and her weekends didn't allow her to recover either.

Recommendations	
1	Add regular ghar ka khaana like poha/upma/paratha, etc., for breakfast; dal rice/roti sabzi + jaggery and ghee for lunch and dinners. (She would cook in two batches per week.)
2	Replace the evening drink with a wholesome snack like rajgira laddoo or a ragi porridge between 4–5 p.m. to avoid cravings later
3	Remove all seeds/powders/kadhas/milk alternatives like oat or almond milk/mock meats and meat alternatives
4	Avoid 'healthy desserts' and instead have a fully loaded dessert of your choice once a week
5	Regulate nap time to 20–30 minutes between 1–3 p.m.
Progress	**In 3 months:**
1	Sugar cravings came down to zero and constipation became nil
2	Pain during periods came down and number of pain killers she needed went from four to zero
3	Had the energy to cook, clean and exercise; reduced hunger pangs and guilt
4	She began to feel normal and not 'dirty' during periods

#6

Who: A small-town techie in his forties, who now leads a unicorn

Ailments: None. But sometimes has stomach pain, disappears on clearing bowels

Goals: Gain weight, better energy and improved gut health

Recalls

5:30 a.m. – woke up	5:30 a.m. – woke up, woke up once at night	Could not clear stomach well last night
6:30 a.m. – athletic greens	6:30 a.m. – red poha, sev	6:30 a.m. – woke up
7–7:50 a.m. – Yoga + weights+ pushups	9:00 a.m. – fruits, uttapam, sambhar	7:00 a.m. – athletic greens
8 a.m. – protein shake (plant-based)	Flight to Bombay	7:30 a.m. – dosa, idli, coffee outside
9 a.m. – soaked dry fruits (7 almonds, 5–6 cranberries, pumpkin, sunflower and chia seeds) + idli sambhar (2)	10:30 a.m. – landed in Bombay, B2B meetings and travel.	10:00 a.m. – walk around 2 kilometres
9 a.m. to 8 p.m. – B2B meetings in office	12:30 p.m. – mushroom soup, Pad Thai, sauted veggies	12:30 p.m. – sushi, avacodo toast
12 p.m. – fruits (papaya)	Lunch meeting	4 p.m. – fruits (banana and grapes)
12:30 p.m. – lunch – brown rice, dal, gobi, peanut chutney	3 p.m. – green tea	
2 p.m. – buttermilk	5 p.m. – sprouted moong chaat	6:30 p.m. – veg clear soup
4 p.m. – fruits (guava and orange)	8 p.m. – dinner meeting:	

7 p.m. – sambhar rice, sauted veggies, 2 eggs (only whites) 9 p.m. – read and meditate 10 p.m. – sleep	beetroot, sweet potato, quinoa Checked into a hotel, crashed 10 p.m. – sleep	7 p.m. – khichdi, moong halwa 8:30 p.m. – reading, in bed, meditation 9:30 p.m. – sleep

Observations: Eats 'fancy' but is not interested in food. Wants to exercise but says he cannot find time. He says his heart wants masala chai but he is living the cold brew dude kind of life. Wants a kachori for breakfast but has settled for athletic greens instead. Craves for chaat and samosa but VC said have sweet potato air fried chips. Only takes food advice from VCs and stops eating eggs when his parents visit.

Recommendations	
1	Replace athletic greens with a banana or raisins or figs on rising
2	Add paratha and sabzi as a breakfast option
3	Remove brown rice, quinoa and have regular rice and dal, roti sabzi and millets of the season
4	Avoid seeds and instead have chutneys
5	Regulate bedtime and cut back on screen time
Progress	**In 3 months:**
1	Improved musculature and lesser aches and pains. Shirts fitted better and he looked less like a lost boy and more like the genius he was (his words)
2	17 reps of regular squats went up to 25 in a minute

3	34 seconds plank went up to 1 minute 14 seconds
4	Gas in the second half of the day settled completely and constipation improved
5	Bowel movement became smoother, and the time taken in the washroom dropped to 5–10 mins from 30–45mins

In Conclusion
A full life

If there is a single sentence that sums up this book it is this – food is the language of life and of love. All my years of work have taught me that PPP is greater than PPP. Pyaar, parivaar and parvarish is infinitely bigger than paisa, position and power. My clients, who come from loving relationships, where families are bonded with affection and where they are raised to have self-esteem, manners and gratitude, do really well with their health. They come from homes where kitchens are still central, where food is still a way to show care, where looking out for each other is default, a way of life.

And money, power, position have nothing to do with this. It is all about love and acceptance, support and acknowledgment, whether the waist is 50 or it is 28. My client's 25-year-old daughter was working with me. When she lost 3 inches in one month, she treated the entire family to pav bhaji and ice cream. She was back from the USA, where she had gained a ton of weight, but no one was waiting for all the weight to come down, they were celebrating progress.

On the other hand, when people have paisa, position and power but lack the other PPP, they lose the same or even more weight or inches, but it doesn't touch them. They don't come from families or environments that have *pehchan* or recognition of their progress. So, they still make progress, but the process is harder on them and on us. Access to people who are invested in our well-being without an agenda, purely out of love, is one of the least celebrated blessings.

The power of pyaar

I worked with Tanya, a smart, savvy, rare woman in her forties who operated out of Singapore and headed the Asia Pacific–Australia region for her company. Rare, because she is one of the only women I know whose mother had preserved her school sports medals. She wasn't an athlete, she never made it to district or state or anything, these were just school medals hung on the wall behind her desk from where she took her calls. Again, a rare sight. Post-pandemic, as my work shifted more online, I saw everything hung on walls, people started having dedicated spaces for calls with good light and some show-off material behind. A golf shot picture, a pic from EBC, a certificate of having completed an executive course from Harvard, etc.

I thought I had seen it all, and then I saw these old medals. She grew up in Mumbai and I recognized the school medals instantly. I think everyone had the same vendor, but I asked to double check. 'Oh! My mom has saved them for all of us three girls. She says it's a reminder that I raised you to work and play.' Wow! *Maaji, charan sparsh*.

I believe, and have seen through my experience, that girls who are celebrated at home, find a way back to nurturing themselves with good food sooner or later. The same was happening with Tanya. She had switched countries, roles, been on the motherhood journey, and with that, through many diets and excessive workouts. At 40-ish, she hit the 'no more bullshit of yo-yo body weight, no more second-guessing every morsel I eat, no more chocolates every night' mode, and that's how I came into the picture.

First things first: we got her to eat but more importantly, she ate without resistance. Women who have received pyaar at home are not resistant to good counsel or to good food. Soon enough, she had the fuel to recover from exercise, push herself harder at work and not snap at her 10-year-old daughter. Within a few months, we were working with her daughter too, a full-time gymnast with the unique distinction of having taught her mom how to do the cartwheel.

Pursuit of purpose

Alright, truth be told, the only bio hack you need is respect for evolution. Ultimately, you and I must vacate our place for those who will come after us and live as gently as possible while we are at it. Evolution is a process that takes the best from us and passes it forward. The best version of us will come only if the current version will make room for it. So honestly, I am not excited about longevity. I find it quite pointless.

Reading glasses will come, if not at 40, then at 50. Walking speed will slow down, if not at 70, then at 80. Deterioration is *pakka*, just like death.

The whole point of looking after the body is to lead a life of joy and purpose. It doesn't protect you from getting sick or dying, but it makes the process easier, or at least more organic. Or, to put it in a different manner, it reduces collateral damage. Let's say (and I sincerely hope this never happens even to my *dushmans*) that you get sick with some condition for which there is no cure or is progressive in nature.

If you are overall fit, not chiselled but eating correctly, exercising regularly, sleeping on time, etc., then your health outcomes are better. You are an easier case not just for the doctor to handle but also for your caregivers. That way, your sickness is only limited to taking a toll on your body, it doesn't damage your family's mental health or at least reduces the toll it takes on them. Less medicines to pop, fewer hospital visits, fewer draining nights, etc.

And if you are blessed with a curable condition, then again it makes it easier on everyone because there are no other complications involved. Harish bhai, the living encyclopaedia on the Himalaya, has been a regular at Iyengar yoga for a few decades and trekking and climbing for over 50–60 years. He has a paunch, but a straight spine and strength in his legs. In his seventies, he went through a hip replacement. Within weeks, he was back to yoga class, and in a few months had returned to trekking.

Good health softens the blow of disease and age, and allows us to pursue our purpose with vigour and strength.

Maturity is knowing that this is all that you want out of your life. And that it doesn't come dressed in six-packs or toned arms.

So I am going to say this: if eating a certain way is commonsensical, don't look towards scientific evidence for approval. Just eat it. Science will catch up, and within your lifetime. Or else we lose a generation to eating sukha roti and avoiding ghee, or eating idli and avoiding coconut chutney. And then through bro-podcasts we rediscover what women have always known: that allowing ourselves the taste, texture, tradition of wholesome food is not just healthy but in tune with the latest in science.

A full life

A full life is not one where you wear the same size of jeans for over twenty years, but the one where you progress with your career, family and other adventures without running out of fuel. Dharma, artha, kama, moksha are important pillars of life. To put it simply: you must be able to pursue the path of dharma, righteousness, through your beliefs, actions, and speech. You must be able to earn wealth of all kinds, emotional, spiritual and even financial. You must be able to pursue pleasures, of art, food and sex. You must be able to keep it together so that your pursuits are not futile; you can live fully, making room for pleasure and pain, without being carried away by them.

They say that everything that can be known is already revealed. The *Kathopanishad* is a dialogue between Yama, the God of Death, and Nachiketa, a young boy. Yama offers Nachiketa endless life, freedom from old age, all the wealth on earth, the company of beautiful women who can sing, dance and entertain, but he isn't lured by it.

'What use is all this wealth?' he asks Yama. 'The senses perceive less over time and all this joy will fade.' (We have all felt that. The first-time shopping at Oxford or Bond Street isn't the same as shopping the third time. Everything external, no matter how exclusive or expensive, fades.) 'I seek that joy which is timeless. That is the only boon I will settle for.' And Yama goes on to tell him the ultimate secret of life and death.

You can read that in good time, but for now, all you need is the fuel to pursue all that you want to in life and to get ripe old with time. Come, let's eat.

Appendices

A. The latest on ...

1. Weight-loss drugs

It's 2025, and 'Glucagon-like peptide-1 receptor agonists (GLP-1RAs)', the likes of Ozempic, Wegovy, Mounjaro, etc., also popularly called the 'weight-loss drugs', will dominate the conversations (for the really rich initially, before cheaper versions flood the market). While there may be a category of people for whom these are beneficial, they are almost being used as a recreational drug. Promoted aggressively by everyone – from medical professionals to influencers – it is already a $50 billion market and is expected to cross $100 billion in next five years.

That there is a long list of side-effects – especially related to the gastrointestinal tract – are just waived off as inconveniences for a greater good. What is the greater good? Weight loss? Most of which is coming from fat-free mass (i.e., muscles, organs, bones, etc.), and that invariably plateaus within 6–12 months as the body makes metabolic adjustments. Not to mention the fact that it bounces back with a vengeance when you stop the medication, which you will at some point due to the side-effects (more than 60 per cent stop).

* 'Ozempic face' has entered the lexicon and describes the wasting and ageing that takes place prominently on the face of those on GLP-1RAs drugs. Similarly, there is an Ozempic butt also.

2. Sugar

1. Don't replace sugar with non-sugar sweeteners, e.g., in your chai, coffee, etc. The WHO, in its latest report on non-sugar sweeteners (NSS),[11] has warned against their use for weight loss or to manage any metabolic disease like diabetes. These include aspartame, saccharin, sucralose, stevia and stevia derivatives.
2. You can safely have regular white sugar in your chai, coffee, sherbets, homemade laddoos, kheer, etc., while staying within recommended sugar limits. The WHO (also USA, Australia, Canada, New Zealand, India) recommends limiting added sugar intake to 5–10 per cent of daily diet. This is about 6–12 tsp per day.
3. What we need to avoid instead are ultra-processed foods (junk foods) like cereals, juices, colas, energy drinks, ketchup, breads, jams, cookies, biscuits, etc.

3. Alcohol

'No amount or kind of alcohol is good for your health. It doesn't matter what alcohol it is – wine, beer, cider or spirits. Drinking alcohol, even a small amount, is damaging to everyone, regardless of age, sex, gender, ethnicity, tolerance for alcohol or lifestyle.'

The above statement is now the official stand of all leading global health organizations including the WHO[12], the *Lancet* and even official government guidelines in countries like Canada. And considering the massive clout of the alcohol industry, it really means the evidence is now impossible to suppress. An aggregate of hundreds of research papers over decades have confirmed beyond doubt that alcohol is toxic. It's now conclusively linked to many types of cancers and mental health issues, along with the already known side-effects of liver damage, high blood sugar, and so on.

As a consumer, make an informed decision regarding alcohol, knowing that a) any one type of alcohol is not better than the other and b) there are no health benefits, only harm.

P.S. Ireland is the first country in the European Union (EU) to ensure that, from 2026, all alcohol products will have comprehensive labelling about health risks from its consumption, including warnings about the risks of developing cancers. In Asia, South Korea is following suit.

4. Social determinants of health

SDOH, as they are known, are the non-medical factors that affect your health. These are conditions in which people are born, live, learn, work, play and age.

Some of the SDOH are:
- *Pincode*: If you live in an area with parks and promenades, you will have access to a neighbourhood where going out for a walk would be an easy and safe choice. Think Bandra West, 400050.
- *Income*: Poverty reduces your chances of access to nutritious food, sanitation and dignity. So everyone having a stable and secure income is not just good for the economy but also good for health.
- *Education*: Access and quality of education has a positive influence on your health. An IPS officer is typically in good shape and a constable, out of shape. The education and income of your mother matters too.
- *Caste, community, class*: Not only do these determine your social mobility but also access to education, jobs and therefore health.
- *Environment*: Air and water pollution outside the house and safety (prevention of domestic violence) inside it.
- *Transportation*: Better mass transport, walkable cities and lesser time sitting in traffic jams, burning fuel and doomscrolling.

SDOH are the reason why conversations should not be reduced to calories, will power, determination to exercise, etc. Because that's really not the complete picture. Everytime your favourite influencer talks about 'excuses', they are overlooking SDOH.

B. One lakh to 12 hajaar

Food	Traditionally eaten as	Appropriated today as
White gourd	– Sabzi – Halwa or petha – Curries with lentils or fish	Juice on empty stomach
Moringa	– Flowers ka sabzi – Sabzi of leaves or their addition to dals and curries – Drumstick in curries and dals	Powder in water on an empty stomach
Cinnamon	– Spice in pulao – Seasoning in pies – Part of masala chai	Cinnamon water in the morning
Jeera	– Part of tadka for khichdi and many sabzis – Added to chaas and buttermilk in cooking – Jeera goli as a digestive	Jeera paani in the morning

Food	Traditionally eaten as	Appropriated today as
Amla	– Achaar and muramba (and chyawanprash) – Sherbet – Amla supari as digestive	Amla shot in the morning
Sattu	– Summer drink in Bihar and parts of North India – Barfis during Teej, shared with all by the Marwari community – Litti in Bihar, popular travel food	Protein shake post workout

C. New junk food

It's easy to tell the junk food; it has ads, jingles, endorsements – almost a recall factor. But then there is the new junk food that is positioning itself like health food. The table below is meant to help you identify both. And for you to know that individual ingredients don't make a food good or bad, it is the processing, shelf life, additives, etc., that are the villains.

If the left column is dominated by large conglomerates, the right one belongs to start-ups who write me emails saying, 'We love your work, join our revolution to make India healthier'. Euphemism for 'Watch us get as big as the conglomerates. Miss out at your own risk.' It is, after all, the fastest-growing category of packaged foods in India.

Irrespective, know that there is no alternative to investing time in learning to cook. And that health cannot be bought off the shelves.

Junk food	'Health-washed' junk food
Sugar-sweetened beverages (SSB) – Colas, juices, caffeinated energy drinks, ready yogurt drinks, etc.	SSB products with zero- or low-calorie sugar substitutes, vitamin enriched or good bacteria versions
Preserves and dressings – Jams, peanut butter, marmalades, ketchup, mustard, mayo, salad dressings, etc.	Low-fat, low-sugar, dairy-free, high protein versions
Chocolates, cakes, ice-creams, biscuits, breakfast cereals, chips and cookies, etc.	Keto, vegan, low-sugar, low-fat, jaggery, gut-friendly, gluten-free, millet, without seed oil versions
Ready to eat or frozen or 2-minute versions – Noodles, pasta, soups, cutlets, hash browns, fries, etc.	Millet, baked, low-sugar, gluten-free, vegan, high-fibre, high-protein versions

Note:

- Health-washing is commonly used by the food industry to position the same junk food as better or healthier (and pricier), by replacing one ingredient in a cocktail of harmful ingredients. E.g., Zero-calorie colas, vegan ice-cream, millet instant noodles, etc.
- Keep the junk food consumption to the bare minimum (a small part of the 20 per cent), regardless of which column you pick from.
- UPF/junk food is addictive in nature, which is why you

want those chips and colas and chocolates, even when you know they are not good for you. Unlike alcohol, there is no 12-step program to help you tackle that.
- The latest studies show that UPFs are not just detrimental to physical but also to mental health.
- The lawsuit on the food industry in the US is being called the tobacco moment for UPFs, one that will make it imperative for the industry to carry a health warning.
- Meantime Robert Kennedy Jr. is vowing to make cola use cane sugar instead of beet. That is like saying vaping is better than smoking. It's the same.

D. Reading list

1. *The Body: A Guide for Occupants* by Bill Bryson, Doubleday, October 2019.
2. 'Randomized Controlled Trials Are Not a Panacea for Diet-Related Research' at https://pmc.ncbi.nlm.nih.gov/articles/ PMC4863268/
3. *The Art of Statistics* by David Spiegelhalter, Pelican, January 2020.
4. 'The Politics of Protein' at https://ipes-food.org/report/the- politics-of-protein/
5. *Why We Sleep: The New Science of Sleep and Dreams* by Matthew Walker, Allen Lane, 3 October 2017.
6. 'Habitually Skipping Breakfast Is Associated with the Risk of Gastrointestinal Cancers: Evidence from the Kailuan Cohort Study' at https://pubmed.ncbi.nlm.nih.gov/36869181/
7. 'Use of BMI Alone Is an Imperfect Clinical Measure' at https://www.ama-assn.org/delivering-care/public-health/ama-use-bmi-alone-imperfect-clinical-measure
8. 'Death of the Calorie' at https://www.economist.com/1843/2019/02/28/death-of-the-calorie

9. *Thinking, Fast and Slow* by Daniel Kahneman, Penguin UL, January 2015.
10. *Ultra-processed People* by Chris Van Tulleken, Penguin, April 2023.
11. 'WHO Advises Not to Use Non-sugar Sweeteners for Weight Control in Newly Released Guideline' at https://www.who.int/news/item/15-05-2023-who-advises-not-to-use-non-sugar-sweeteners-for-weight-control-in-newly-released-guideline
12. 'No Level of Alcohol Consumption Is Safe for Our Health' at https://www.who.int/europe/news/item/04-01-2023-no-level-of-alcohol-consumption-is-safe-for-our-health

A Note on the Author

Rujuta Diwekar is India's leading public health advocate and amongst the most followed nutritionists globally. Her books have sold more than 1.75 million copies and her videos have been viewed more than 300 million times. Her clear and simple message to eat local, seasonal, and traditional, has redefined the discourse on health and wellness, nudging it away from diet trends and towards sustainable well-being of people and the planet.

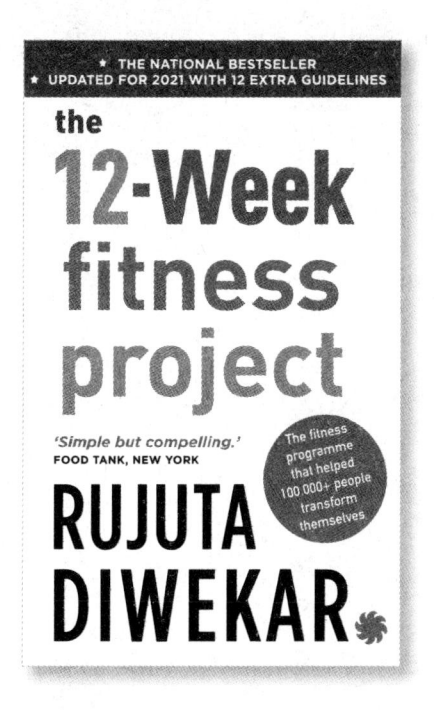

The 12-Week Fitness Project

Lose inches. Gain health. Sleep better. In just 12 weeks.

Want to get fit but don't know how to start? Let India's #1 nutritionist and health advocate Rujuta Diwekar help you. In this groundbreaking book, based on the '12-week fitness project', one of the world's largest and most successful public health projects, she will guide you step by step, giving you one simple guideline to follow each week.

By the end of three months you will have transformed your habits in twelve crucial ways. The result? You'll find you have lost inches and have better sleep and energy levels, lesser acidity, bloating and sweet cravings and reduced PMS and period pain.

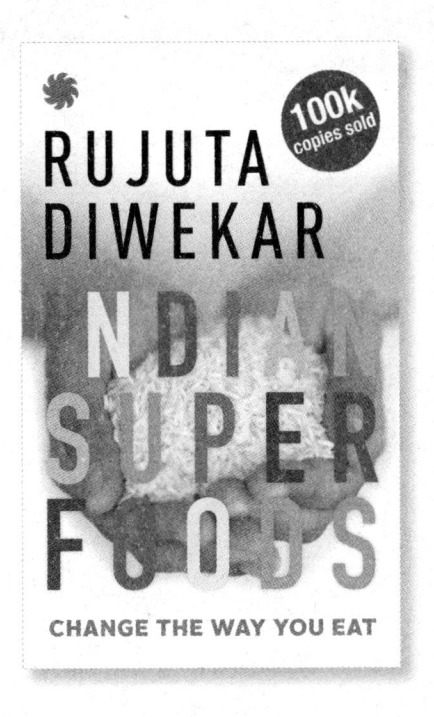

Indian Superfoods

Forget about acacia seeds and goji berries. The secret foods for health, vitality and weight loss lie in our own kitchens and backyards. From aphrodisiacs to fertility boosters, fat burners to mind calmers, top nutritionist Rujuta Diwekar talks you through the ten Indian superfoods that will completely transform you.